- Do you find t[...]

- Do you suffer [...] sexual dysfunction, yet worry about the potential dangers of using a prescription drug, such as Viagra?

- Would you like to slow the effects of aging—on both the mind and body?

- Or are you simply looking to sharpen your concentration and memory?

IF YOU ANSWERED "YES" TO ANY
OF THESE QUESTIONS,
LEARN THE SECRETS OF ONE OF
THE MOST POPULAR HERBAL
SUPPLEMENTS ON THE MARKET.

LEARN THE
SECRETS OF GINKGO

SECRETS
of
GINKGO

WINIFRED CONKLING

St. Martin's Paperbacks

Author's Note

This book is for informational purposes only. It is not intended to take the place of medical advice from a trained medical professional. Readers are advised to consult a physician or other qualified health professional regarding treatment of all of their health problems or before acting on any of the information or advice in this book. The fact that an organization or Web site is mentioned in this book as a source of information or herbs does not mean that the author or publisher recommends it.

Contents

CONTENTS

Introduction

The ginkgo is one of the oldest species of tree in the world, dating back to the time when dinosaurs roamed the earth. More recently, it has been planted as an ornamental tree both for its beauty and heartiness. The ginkgo biloba tree is strong enough to withstand assaults by insects and many plant diseases; it even survived the atomic blast at Hiroshima.

Although ginkgo has been used as a medicinal herb in Asia for several thousand years, it has only been "discovered" as an important medicinal herb in the United States in the last thirty years or so. Today ginkgo is one of the leading prescription medicines in France and Germany and is one of the most popular herbs in the United States.

Ginkgo's rapid rise to popularity reflects its effectiveness at improving circulation, boosting memory, treating heart disease, and more. Researchers have shown that some of the active ingredients in ginkgo help to dilate the arteries, veins, and capillaries and to improve peripheral blood flow, resulting in improved circulation. Improved circulation means that more nourishing oxygen reaches the entire body, especially the brain. When life-giving oxygen reaches the brain, it helps in the treatment of short-term memory loss, tinnitus (ringing in the ears), senility, and other problems caused by vascular disease.

This book will let you in on the secrets of ginkgo biloba and introduce you to the many health benefits attributed to the herb. *Secrets of Ginkgo* is divided into three main sections:

- Part 1, "Understanding Ginkgo," outlines the history and folklore surrounding the herb. It also describes the types of ginkgo and explains how the active ingredients work to make the herb effective.

- Part 2, "The Healing Power of Ginkgo," describes how the herb can be used to enhance brain function, improve circulation, overcome impotence, protect vision and hearing, and to aid other medical problems.

- Part 3, "Using Ginkgo," offers advice on buying and using the herb; it also provides information on when and how to use ginkgo to improve your overall health.

The information in this book is based on both folk medicine and contemporary research. It includes the knowledge that has been passed down for thousands of years by herbalists experienced in the use of ginkgo as well as the findings of carefully controlled studies that have been published in peer-reviewed medical journals. This comprehensive approach to understanding ginkgo will enable you to appreciate the special qualities of this unique herb and choose how you use ginkgo to enhance your overall health and well-being.

A SUMMARY OF WHAT GINKGO CAN DO FOR YOU

- **Ginkgo increases blood flow to the brain.** This increased blood flow helps boost memory, concentration, and mental functioning. It also helps to prevent confusion, headaches, and depression caused by poor blood and oxygen circulation to the brain.

- **Ginkgo improves blood flow to the extremities.** This makes ginkgo very effective in the treatment of peripheral vascular disease, which can cause poor circulation to the legs. In severe cases, peripheral vascular disease can weaken the legs to the point that walking becomes difficult.

- **Ginkgo is a powerful antioxidant, or free-radical scavenger.** The herb helps prevent tissue damage caused by exposure to excessive sunlight, radiation, pesticides, and herbicides.

- **Ginkgo improves blood vessel tone and makes the capillaries more permeable.** This strengthens the entire cardiovascular system and allows for improved transfer of oxygen to the cells.

- **Ginkgo inhibits the excessive immune response responsible for allergies, asthma, and skin problems, among others.**

- **Ginkgo protects hearing.** It is helpful in the treatment of tinnitus, vertigo (dizziness), and hearing loss.

- **Ginkgo improves vision and helps to prevent some eye problems associated with aging.** The herb helps prevent free-radical damage to the retinas, which can cause macular degeneration and other vision problems.

- **Ginkgo protects the linings of the nerves against damage.** This can help in the treatment of multiple sclerosis.

- **Ginkgo improves the uptake and utilization of oxygen and glucose (sugar) in the body.** This improves brain function, helps control diabetes, and helps the body manage stress.

- **Ginkgo helps maintain equilibrium and balance.**

PART ONE

Understanding Ginkgo

CHAPTER 1

A Natural Wonder: The History of Ginkgo

Ginkgo biloba has earned the name "the living fossil" as ginkgo trees thrived during prehistoric times, growing wild throughout the world. During the last ice age, however, the ginkgo tree almost became extinct; it survived only in Asia. About 1,000 years ago, ginkgos were planted as ornamental trees in Japanese monastery gardens, where they were nurtured by monks.

The ginkgo tree has been around for more than 200 million years, and perhaps as long as 280 million years. It has been used as a medicinal herb for more than 5,000 years. Ginkgo's longevity extends to the plant itself. Some ginkgo trees have been known to live well over 1,000 years.

The ginkgo tree is a native of southeastern

China, although it is grown as a popular ornamental tree throughout the world. A decorative ginkgo tree was planted in the Botanical Garden in Utrecht, Holland, in 1727 after being brought from Japan. The ginkgo tree made its way to the United States in 1784, when it was planted in William Hamilton's garden in Philadelphia. Since that time has become a popular ornamental tree in urban areas; it grows in many parks and gardens in London and New York City.

GETTING TO KNOW GINKGO

Ginkgo is a deciduous conifer (cone-bearing plant) with separate male and female types. Male flowers look something like cattails (they're called catkins); the female bears a plumlike fruit (sometimes called nuts). The male flowers produce free-swimming reproductive pollen cells, which is typical of ferns and cycads (tropical plants such as palms) but not of conifers.

The tree has rootlike growths that hang down from its branches. The Chinese call these zhong ru, or stalactites, while the Japanese call them chichi, or breasts. According to Japanese folklore, a particular ginkgo tree planted over the grave of an Emperor's wet nurse has special powers. The tree—which has many "breasts"—is said to provide breast milk to any woman who prays to the tree for the ability to nurse her children.

The male pollen is carried by the wind to the female tree, which produces ovules that, when fertilized, develop into yellowish seeds about one inch long. These seeds consist of a large silvery nut surrounded by a fleshy outer fruit; when ripe the fruit has the distinct—and unpleasant—odor of rancid butter. The odor of the ginkgo fruit is impossible to wash out of fabric. The fruit also can cause people to break out in a poison ivy–like rash; see Chapter 8 for more information. In the United States, the fruit is considered a foul-smelling nuisance, but in China, Japan, and other Asian cultures it often is considered a delicacy. For centuries, the Chinese and Japanese have roasted the seeds and used them as a digestive aid and a way to prevent drunkenness. Today the seeds are dyed red and served at weddings and parties involving the use of alcohol. In New York City, Chinese women go to Central Park to gather ginkgo seeds as they drop. (Of course, they wear gloves to protect their skin from the rash-producing fruit.)

APPRECIATING GINKGO

Ginkgo has been a staple of Chinese herbal medicines for thousands of years, being recommended for coughs, asthma, allergies, as well as circulatory disorders, memory loss, and symptoms associated with aging. As early as 2800 B.C. ginkgo was used to re-

---

THE NAME GAME

The name "ginkgo biloba" is derived from the Japanese word *ginkyo* and the Chinese word *yinkuo*, which mean "silver apricot." The leaves have two lobes, giving the plant its second name, "biloba."

It is also called the kew or maidenhair tree because its leaves look like the fronds of the maidenhair fern. Some botanists consider the ginkgo the "missing link" between ferns and flowering plants.

---

store memory and ease breathing problems. It is one of the ingredients in the traditional Hindu medicine known as soma. It was not widely used for medicinal purposes in the United States, however, until the 1980s, when isolating the essential components of ginkgo became technically feasible. Scientists isolated two main groups of substances—the flavonoids (or antioxidants) and the terpenes (or anticlotting agents). In general, most researchers have focused on ginkgo's ability to improve blood circulation.

Within a decade, ginkgo has become one of the most popular herbs sold in the United States. It seems that every few months a new study is completed that demonstrates ginkgo's healing benefits, making it still more popular. Ginkgo has earned a reputation as an herb that can promote youth and longevity, largely because it helps to improve brain function.

Today ginkgo has been the subject of more than 300 published reports in the West. These studies have confirmed ginkgo's amazing healing powers, especially its ability to improve circulation. Because good circulation is essential for all bodily functions, every system can benefit from ginkgo therapy. Part 2 summarizes the ways ginkgo can be used in the management of specific health problems.

CHAPTER 2

How Ginkgo Works: The Active Ingredients

People have used ginkgo biloba and other medicinal herbs in healing for thousands of years, but only recently have scientists begun to understand how they work. Carefully controlled clinical studies have demonstrated ginkgo's healing properties, but understanding the complexities of how herbal remedies work in the body is extraordinarily difficult. Ginkgo and other herbs contain hundreds of chemicals, many of which work together synergistically to produce certain biological effects.

In their research on ginkgo, researchers have isolated certain active ingredients thought to be the most important in healing. The researchers have attempted to identify the physiological properties assigned to each of the constituents by comparing plants with similar ingredients and looking for shared characteristics. (For example, two plants with similar ingredients may both thin the blood, so researchers may examine whether the shared ingredient affects clotting time when used in isolation.) This research helps herbalists determine which active ingredients contribute to a given biological effect.

Ginkgo has two main types of active ingredients, flavone glycosides and terpene lactones. For the herb to be most effective, it must have the proper balance of these ingredients.

FLAVONE GLYCOSIDES

Flavone glycosides are a type of flavonoids, or antioxidants, found in a number of plants and fruits, especially citrus fruits. In addition to working as antioxidants, these compounds strengthen the capillary walls, reduce inflammation, and help prevent bruising. (Antioxidants are discussed in greater detail later in this chapter.) The flavone glycosides include quercetin, kaempferol, and isorhamnetin. The optimal level is 22 to 27 percent of the active ingredients; check the label of the product you are buying to be sure it contains this amount of flavone glycosides.

TERPENE LACTONES

Terpene lactones are unique to the ginkgo tree; they include bilobalides and ginkgolides A, B, C, and J. These terpene lactones help to thin the blood and prevent blood clots. They improve blood circulation to the brain and help the body use glucose (sugar) more effectively. They also protect the nerve cells from damage during periods of oxygen deprivation. The powerful ginkgolides are not well understood, but they are given credit for many of ginkgo's healing attributes. Some researchers believe that the ginkgolides achieve these impressive healing feats by interfering with a chemical found in the body called PAF (platelet-activating factor). PAF has been implicated in cases of graft rejection, asthma, and other immune disorders. By inhibiting PAF in the blood, ginkgo helps to boost circulation. The optimal level is 5 to 7 percent of these active ingredients; check the label of the product you are buying to be sure it contains this amount of terpene lactones. Ginkgo also includes minor organic acids such as hydroxykynurenic acid, pyrocatchuic acid, kynurenic acid, vanilla acid, and hydroxy benzoic acid.

GINKGO AS AN ANTIOXIDANT

Antioxidants such as ginkgo help to decrease cell damage caused by free radicals, which are highly reactive molecules that contain unpaired electrons. Free radicals are a by-product of certain metabolic processes; they enter the body with food and air pollution; and they also are by-products of radiation. In the body, these free radicals are unstable; they randomly damage other cells by trying to steal electrons away from their neighbors. Over time the free radicals damage cells by destroying the cells' genetic material or outer membrane.

The results of oxidation can be devastating. A number of disorders have been linked to free-radical damage. According to some researchers, the evidence is mounting that most diseases at some point in their development are related to tissue injury caused by free-radical reaction. Some conditions associated with free-radical damage include: premature aging, alcoholism, Alzheimer's disease, brain edema, cancer, senile dementia, demyelination, head trauma, heart attack, Parkinson's disease, retinal damage, stroke, spinal cord damage, inflammation, hardening of the arteries, intestinal ischemia (lack of oxygen to the organs), and pancreatitis.

GINKGO BY ANY OTHER NAME

Unlike other herbs with scores of nicknames based on regional folklore, ginkgo has only a few names. Most make reference to the tree's fan-shaped leaves. The names include:

- Buddha's fingernail
- Duck foot
- Fly-moth leaf
- Maidenhair tree

Chinese herbalists refer to it as

- Fei-o-hsich
- Fu chi-chia
- Kung-sun shu
- Ya-chiao-pan

Ginkgo, as well as other antioxidants such as vitamin A, the B-complex vitamins, selenium, and vitamin E, helps to reduce the number of potentially damaging free radicals

GINKGO GROWN IN THE LAB

Mother Nature's work is so complex that researchers have only begun to isolate and research the many chemical constituents of ginkgo and other herbs. While no one can replicate the herbal masterpiece known as ginkgo, researchers at Harvard University in 1988 were able to synthesize one of the ginkgo's most important constituents, ginkgolide B.

By creating a laboratory version of this ingredient, it can be tested as a possible remedy for a number of different medical problems, including asthma, Alzheimer's disease, and circulatory disorders. It may also prove useful as a substitute for drugs used to prevent organ rejection after transplants. Research is currently underway to investigate medical applications for synthetic ginkgolide B.

in the body. The antioxidants "scavenge" for free radicals, cleaning them up and rendering them harmless by donating to these cells an extra electron. A number of studies have demonstrated ginkgo's effectiveness as a potent free-radical scavenger.

PART TWO

The Healing Power of Ginkgo

CHAPTER 3

Ginkgo and the Brain

Ginkgo biloba is probably best known for its ability to enhance brain function, to improve memory and concentration, and to help reverse the ravages of Alzheimer's disease and senile dementia. Ginkgo achieves these impressive results by improving blood circulation to the brain, which is particularly sensitive to oxygen deprivation. The brain needs a steady supply of oxygen and glucose, both of which depend on adequate blood circulation. Healthy, robust blood flow is particularly important in today's environment, where stress, smoking, alcohol, and other factors conspire to compromise alertness, recall, and overall brain functioning.

When it comes to improving blood circulation to the brain, ginkgo stands alone.

As discussed later in the chapter, studies have shown that ginkgo is more effective than other herbs or synthetic drugs at enhancing blood flow. In addition, the herb has been found to improve electrical transmission in the nerves, speeding the rate at which the brain can process information.

Ginkgo is also a powerful antioxidant, which is particularly important in the brain. The brain cell membranes consist of a high percentage of unsaturated fatty acids, making them especially vulnerable to free-radical damage and oxygen deprivation.

ALZHEIMER'S DISEASE AND SENILE DEMENTIA

One of the advantages of growing older is that we accumulate the wisdom and precious memories of a lifetime. Unfortunately, Alzheimer's disease and senile dementia can rob us of this knowledge, which is part of what makes us who we are. Some four million older Americans—including two out of three nursing-home patients—suffer from Alzheimer's disease or senile dementia. When the condition was first described by a German neurologist in 1907, Alzheimer's disease was considered a rare disorder, but today it is regarded as the most common cause of senile dementia. A 1989 study in the *Journal of the American Medical Association* found that 10.3 percent of people over age sixty-five had "probable Alzheimer's disease."

With Alzheimer's disease, the body malfunctions and gradually destroys the nerve cells in several key areas of the brain. As the disease progresses, the nerve fibers around the hippocampus—the brain's memory center—become crossed and knotted; these neurofibrillary tangles make it impossible to store or retrieve information. In addition to this internal short circuit, the brain also experiences a drop in the concentration of neurotransmitting substances, which further breaks down the body's communications network.

Alzheimer's usually develops gradually. The symptoms often include memory loss and loss of the intellectual skills needed to work and socialize normally. A person may experience confusion, difficulty in communicating, trouble finding the right word, impaired judgment, disorientation, and/or changes in personality and behavior.

Dementia (or senile dementia) refers to general mental deterioration, including memory loss, moodiness, irritability, personality changes, childish behavior, difficulty communicating, and inability to concentrate. Alzheimer's disease is a type of dementia. Other causes of dementia include Huntington's, Parkinson's, Pick's, and Creutzfeld-Jacob diseases.

Alzheimer's disease, dementia, and other progressive losses of mental functioning shouldn't be considered a normal or inevitable part of the aging process. These conditions are signs that something has gone wrong. In a healthy person, intellectual performance can remain relatively uncompromised well into the nineties, provided the mind remains stimulated through learning. Most older people do not lose a significant portion of their mental functioning; if they do, it is usually the result of a physical problem, such as a stroke.

Unfortunately, when it comes to Alzheimer's disease and dementia, we do not fully understand the disease process or what triggers it, although there does appear to be a hereditary link. What we do know is that the brains of Alzheimer's patients tend to contain high levels of aluminum, calcium, silicon, and sulfur.

Ginkgo has been shown to be useful in the treatment of Alzheimer's disease, senility, dementia, and other forms of age-related mental dysfunction, especially when it is used during the early stages of these diseases. In many cases these forms of mental impairment are caused by insufficient blood flow and oxygen supply to the brain cells. The brain is literally starved for oxygen, resulting in short-term memory loss, vertigo, headache, and depression. Ginkgo can help to delay or reverse some of the problems associated with these diseases. Consider the evidence:

- A double-blind study of fifty people with moderate senile dementia found that ginkgo could improve mental functioning. In the study, conducted in Paris, fifty people were given either ginkgo or a placebo (sugar pill); those who received ginkgo experienced significant improvement in their mood and sociability.

- In another study, researchers gave 120 milligrams ginkgo extract to 112 geriatric patients who suffered from inadequate cerebral blood flow. These patients experienced a significant reversal in symptoms, demonstrating that many of the so-called age-related mental disorders may be caused by reduced blood flow to the brain rather than damage to the nerve cells themselves.

- In 1997 researchers completed a study of 200 people who had suffered from dementia caused by either Alzheimer's disease or multiple ministrokes. Study participants were given 120 milligrams ginkgo extract daily for six months to one year; those who took the herb scored higher on several tests of mental performance and social behavior compared to members of the control group who took a placebo. Researchers found that ginkgo slowed mental decline and that about one out of five people who took the herb may have experienced some slight improvement in their overall mental health.

- German researchers conducted a three-month, double-blind study of forty people (ages sixty to eighty) who had been diagnosed with primary degenerative dementia. Half the study participants received 120 milligrams ginkgo a day, while the others were given a placebo. The researchers found that the people taking the ginkgo were more alert, had a more positive outlook, and scored higher on other measures of mental health compared to those in the control group, who showed no improvement.

- In 1975 French researchers examined the potential benefits of using ginkgo to treat impaired blood flow to the brain. As part of the three-month study, half of the sixty study participants were given 120 milligrams ginkgo biloba extract daily and the others were given a placebo. The researchers tested the participants in the first part of the study to get a baseline for their levels of dizziness, headache, and mental functioning. Follow-up exams at the end of the study found that the ginkgo group had a 79 percent improvement in these tests, compared to a 21 percent improvement in the placebo group.

GINKGO AND MEMORY

A number of studies have demonstrated ginkgo's ability to enhance memory. This quality may make ginkgo of particular use to epileptics who take anticonvulsant drugs, which can impair memory function. More research is needed, but some scientists speculate that ginkgo may help to block inappropriate electrical impulses in the brains of people with epilepsy, which could reduce the number of seizures while at the same time improving memory.

Several studies have demonstrated ginkgo's ability to enhance memory.

- Ginkgo has been shown to improve short-term memory. In a double-blind study, one group of healthy young women was given a ginkgo extract, and the other was given a placebo. On a memory test, the reaction time in the women who had taken the ginkgo improved significantly. Electroencephalogram (EEG) tracings of the women's brains also showed increased brain-wave activity in the women taking ginkgo.

- Researchers in London examined the benefits of ginkgo on thirty-one patients over the age of fifty who showed signs of memory impairment. Half the study participants were given 120 milligrams ginkgo daily; the others took a placebo. The participants were examined and tested at the beginning of the study, at twelve weeks, and at twenty-four weeks of treatment. The people taking the ginkgo showed significantly superior improvement in memory compared to those in the placebo group. EEGs of all the study participants also showed improved brain activity in the ginkgo group.

- Of nine double-blind studies measuring the effect of ginkgo on cerebral impairment due to circulation problems in the brain, the overall improvement rate ranged from 44 to 92 percent, compared to 14 to 44 percent for the people in the placebo groups. The studies lasted from five weeks to twelve months.

TEN TRICKS TO IMPROVE YOUR MEMORY

While ginkgo can help improve the circulation in your brain and thus improve memory, other tricks can help to improve recall. Having a good memory is like having a well-organized desk—the information is there, and you know how to get your hands on it. By practicing these techniques while using ginkgo, you can enhance your memory and information retrieval systems even faster than using ginkgo alone.

1. **Pay attention**. It's impossible to remember something when you're experiencing sensory overload. Focus your attention on one thing at a time so that your brain will know how to file it away.

2. **Make a mental picture**. If you want to remember a name, take a "snapshot" of the person in context, paying special attention to what they are wearing, how they speak, and any other details that seem important to you. Try to focus on something distinctive about the person.

3. **Make up a rhyme.** To remember some-one's name, make up a jingle or rhyme asso-ciated with the name, such as "Anna Banana in a yellow bandanna."

4. **Write it down.** If you want to remember something, take notes. The process of writing will help you recall the information—and you will have written notes to refer to if, despite your efforts, you forget.

5. **Say it again . . . and again.** If you want to remember someone's name, repeat it out loud at least three times during your conver-sation. "Nice to meet you, Jonathan. I like the name Jonathan. I have a brother named Jona-than." If you want to remember something you read, discuss the text with someone else.

6. **Review to remember.** If you want to remember something, review it soon after you have heard or read it. If you're concerned about forgetting people's names, reviewing the names of possible guests at a party or social gathering beforehand may prove helpful.

7. **Cross-reference your files**. Expanding on the idea that memories are stored in files, you can enhance your retrieval system by con-sciously filing a memory in several places. For example, if you want to remember that

Roger's new baby is named Ella, you might want to remember that Roger's other child is named Hannah; both names have two syllables; both children have blond hair; as a child, you knew kids named both Ella and Hannah. Now, when you need to recall the names of Roger's children, you have several paths of retrieval—childhood friends, two-syllable names, girls with blond hair, and so forth.

8. **Make it easy on yourself.** It's not cheating to use lists, calendars, pocket computers, and other tools to help you remember things.

9. **Form consistent habits.** You won't need to remember where you put the car keys if you put them in the same place every time you come in the door. Likewise, it's easy to find the car in the parking lot if you always park in the same general area when you go to the mall.

10. **Use gimmicks.** Try mnemonic devices to remember a list of items. For example, HOMES can be used to recall the Great Lakes: *H*uron, *O*ntario, *M*ichigan, *E*rie, and *S*uperior. Or, to remember how to spell the word "arithmetic," you can make up a sentence, such as: A rat in the house may eat the ice cream.

PREVENTING ALZHEIMER'S AND SENILE DEMENTIA

Scientists do not understand fully the causes of Alzheimer's disease and senile dementia, but many experts believe that aluminum in the body can contribute to its development. To minimize your exposure to aluminum, avoid certain products (such as douches, feminine hygiene products, deodorants, and antidandruff shampoos containing aluminum), and medications (such as antacids, some buffered aspirins, and antidiarrheal medications). At one time people were cautioned to avoid aluminum cookware, but research has shown that aluminum from cookware does not affect overall health.

OTHER HERBS USEFUL FOR BRAIN ENHANCEMENT

While ginkgo stands out as one of the best herbs for improved brain functioning, several other herbs also show promise. These include:

• **Alfalfa (Medicago sativa):** Alfalfa also helps to improve blood circulation in the brain, which helps to oxygenate the cells and promotes better brain functioning.

• **Club moss (Huperzia serrata):** Chinese healers have long prescribed tea brewed from Oriental club moss to reverse memory loss in older people.

• **Garlic (Allium sativum):** Animal research has shown that garlic appears to slow down brain deterioration of laboratory rats with Alzheimer's disease.

FOR MORE INFORMATION

If you or a loved one experience symptoms of Alzheimer's disease that do not respond to treatment with ginkgo, consider requesting additional information from your doctor or from one of the following organizations:

Alzheimer's Disease Society
2 West 45th Street, Room 1703
New York, NY 10036
(212) 719-4744

**Alzheimer's Disease and Related
Disorders Association**
919 North Michigan Avenue, Suite 100
Chicago, IL 60611
(312) 335-8700
(800) 272-3900

**The American Journal of Alzheimer's
Care and Related Disorders**
470 Boston Post Road
Weston, MA 02193
(617) 899-2702

CHAPTER 4

Ginkgo and the Heart and Circulatory System

Your heart and circulatory system feed every cell in your body with life-giving oxygen. This complex 12,400-mile network of arteries, veins, and blood vessels circulates blood from your heart to the farthest reaches of your body. In a healthy adult, the heart beats about 100,000 times a day, pumping the equivalent of more than 4,000 gallons of blood. That's an impressive accomplishment—one that underscores the importance of maintaining a well-tuned heart and circulatory system.

But all too often the system fails. Most of the problems arise from malfunctions of the central pump, the heart, or from damage to the blood vessels. Heart attacks, atherosclerosis, congestive heart failure, strokes, and other circulatory diseases claim about one million lives a year in the United States. In addition, a huge number of Americans— more than sixty-three million—live with some form of heart or blood vessel disease. Heart disease kills more Americans than any other ailment.

Although the risk of heart attack and cardiovascular disease increases with age, about one-fifth of the deaths occur among people under age sixty-five. Fortunately, many of these deaths can be prevented by lifestyle changes and by avoiding or minimizing the factors that raise the risk of cardiovascular disease.

HEART ATTACK

The heart is a muscle, and like any other muscle, it needs oxygen to stay alive. When all or part of the heart muscle dies due to a lack of oxygen, it is called a heart attack, or myocardial infarction. Each year more than 1.5 million Americans suffer heart attacks, and about one out of three of them dies.

Many heart attacks are caused by blood clots. When blood flows through an artery of the heart that has been narrowed by atherosclerosis, it slows down and tends to clot. Large enough clots cut off the blood supply to the portion of the heart muscle below them, and that part of the heart muscle begins to die.

Heart attack can also occur when the heartbeat becomes irregular. In severe cases, this condition, known as arrhythmia, can prevent sufficient blood from reaching the heart muscle.

ATHEROSCLEROSIS

"Hardening of the arteries," or atherosclerosis, involves the gradual buildup of fatty deposits, or plaque, in the arteries. The deposits narrow the arteries, reducing the blood supply to the heart and increasing the likelihood that a blood clot will clog up an arterial pathway and cause a heart attack.

Atherosclerosis is a three-step process. First, the arteries develop tiny tears due to the heart's powerful contractions, especially if the person has high blood pressure. Next, cholesterol in the blood sticks to these tears and slowly hardens into plaque. This causes the arteries to become less flexible. Finally, these deposits narrow the arterial passages, reducing the blood supply to the heart muscle and other parts of the body.

The heart muscle is so efficient at extracting oxygen from the blood that many people develop severe coronary disease before any symptoms appear. In fact, the vessels can be 70 to 90 percent blocked before any symptoms occur—and often a heart attack is the first warning sign that something is wrong.

When it involves the coronary arteries, atherosclerosis causes heart attacks. When atherosclerosis blocks blood flow to the brain, it causes stroke. And when it affects the arteries of the legs, it causes peripheral vascular disease.

CONGESTIVE HEART FAILURE

When the heart has been damaged and can no longer pump efficiently but has not failed outright, a person is suffering from congestive heart failure. When this occurs, the kidneys respond to the reduced blood circulation by retaining salt and water in the body, which causes the heart muscle to have to work even harder.

Congestive heart failure can affect either the right or left side of the heart. The left side pumps oxygen-rich blood from the lungs to the rest of the body. The right side of the heart pumps oxygen-depleted blood back from the body to the lungs, where oxygen is replenished. When the left side of the heart is damaged, the blood backs up in the lungs, causing wheezing and shortness of breath (even during rest), fatigue, sleep disturbances, and a dry, hacking, nonproductive cough when lying down. When the right side of the heart is damaged, the blood collects in the legs and liver, causing swollen feet and ankles, swollen neck veins, pain below the ribs, fatigue, and lethargy.

STROKE

A stroke is like a heart attack in the brain. Just as a part of the heart dies when deprived of oxygen during a heart attack, so a part of the brain dies when deprived of oxygen during a stroke. There are three different types of stroke:

- A **thrombotic** stroke occurs when an artery in the brain is blocked by a clot or atherosclerosis.

- An **embolic** stroke occurs when a small clot (known as an embolus) forms elsewhere in the body and moves to the brain, where it lodges in an artery and blocks the flow of blood.

- A **hemorrhagic** stroke occurs when an artery in the brain ruptures, usually due to high blood pressure. While hemorrhagic strokes are less common—causing only about 20 percent of all strokes—they are much more lethal, causing about 50 percent of all stroke-related deaths.

After a stroke, the person loses the bodily functions associated with the part of the brain that was destroyed. Symptoms of a stroke include slurred speech or loss of speech; sudden severe headache; double vision or blindness; sudden weakness or loss of sensation in the limbs; or loss of consciousness. These symptoms can occur over a period of a few minutes or hours, and they can occur on one side of the body or both.

Stroke is the nation's third leading cause of death and the leading cause of adult disability. Experts estimate that as many as 80 percent of all strokes can be prevented either through changes in lifestyle or through the use of drugs to control high blood pressure and the tendency to form clots.

GETTING TO THE HEART OF THE MATTER

Ginkgo has a profound effect on the cardiovascular system because it dilates the veins and arteries, which improves blood circulation. In addition, it thins the blood, reducing the likelihood of developing blood clots. The bioflavonoids in ginkgo allow the herb to scavenge free radicals in the body, protecting the heart and vessels from cellular damage. These bioflavonoids also provide protection to blood vessels against the damaging effect of plaque buildup.

Ginkgo also inhibits the clumping of blood platelets, which can contribute to cardiovascular disease. When platelets stick to the walls of blood vessels, clots and blockages can form, possibly resulting in heart attack or stroke. Ginkgo contains ginkgolides, compounds that inhibit platelet-activating factor (PAF), which controls the formation of clots.

CONSIDER THE EVIDENCE

A number of studies have confirmed the benefits of using ginkgo in the management and prevention of cardiovascular disease.

- A 1965 study reported that ginkgo biloba extract lowered blood pressure and dilated, or expanded, the peripheral blood vessels and capillaries in ten patients with cardiovascular disease.

- In 1972 researchers compared the use of ginkgo extract with other vasodilators (hydrogenated alkaloids of ergot, acetylcholine chloride, and sodium nicotinate) in people with varying degrees of vascular disease. The researchers found that the ginkgo extract was as effective as the other vasodilators, and it yielded more consistent results.

- A 1977 study looked at the impact of ginkgo extract on the cerebral blood flow in twenty patients, ages sixty-two to eighty-five, who were diagnosed with cerebral circulatory insufficiency due to hardening of the arteries. The study participants received ginkgo both orally and by injection for fifteen days. The researchers found that blood flow in the brain increased dramatically in fifteen of the twenty patients.

- Another 1977 study found that ginkgo extract was very effective in treating peripheral vascular disease. The researchers found that 65 percent of the study participants who had arterial leg disease improved, compared to 22 percent in the control group. In addition, study participants reported improved circulation to the legs, a lessening of impotence, and the clearing of some skin conditions. A further analysis showed that the ginkgo was 100 percent effective in treating people with Grade II lower limb arterial inflammation; there was also a 33 percent response among people with Raynaud's disease (a circulatory problem in the fingers and toes).

- Another study found that ginkgo was as effective as several prescription medicines used to treat arterial disease. Ginkgo extract (160 milligrams per day) was given orally to thirty-eight people with peripheral vascular disease. The six-month study found that ginkgo was more effective than 600 milligrams buflomedial (a prescription drug used to treat the condition) and as effective as 1,200 milligrams pentoxifylline (another drug used to treat the same condition).

- In 1984 a six-month, double-blind study examined the efficacy of ginkgo extract in patients with peripheral arterial insufficiency. There was a marked improvement in walking without pain and increased blood flow to lower limbs in the group that received the ginkgo.

- Ginkgo has been show to increase blood flow in the capillaries and small vessels as well as in the larger ones. German researchers in Hamburg in 1992 studied the circulation of blood in the capillaries of ten participants. The results showed a 57 percent increase in blood flow through the capillaries of the fingers one hour after study participants took oral doses of ginkgo.

- Several studies have shown that ginkgo helps the heart contract more effectively in times of stress by reducing the formation of free radicals. This protective effect can help prevent damage to heart muscle that may become oxygen deprived.

AN OUNCE OF PREVENTION

The major risk factors for heart disease and circulatory problems include smoking, high blood pressure, obesity, high blood cholesterol levels, and a family history of the disease. There are steps you can take to reduce many of these risks.

- **Stop smoking.** Smoking constricts the arteries, raises blood pressure, increases arterial tearing, speeds atherosclerosis, and reduces oxygen levels in the blood. Smokers have two to four times the risk of heart attack as nonsmokers, and their heart attacks are more likely to be fatal. But there is hope: A decade after quitting, a former pack-a-day smoker has almost the same heart attack risk as if he or she had never smoked.

- **Exercise to keep your arteries strong and flexible**. Aerobic exercise helps prevent cardiovascular disease by lowering low-density-lipoprotein (LDL) cholesterol levels and raising high-density lipoprotein (HDL) cholesterol levels, reducing blood pressure, keeping weight down, burning fat, lowering blood-sugar levels, and boosting relaxation. People who exercise regularly are about half as likely as sedentary people to have a heart attack. Furthermore, people who exercise as part of their rehabilitation after a heart attack have a 25 percent reduction in the number of second attacks.

- **Maintain a healthy body weight**. Excess body fat increases blood pressure and adds stress to the heart and circulatory system. People who maintain their ideal body weight are 35 to 55 percent less likely to have a heart attack than those who are obese (20 percent or more above their ideal weight).

- **Become more aware of your anger, anxiety, and fear**. These negative emotions trigger the release of adrenaline and increase blood pressure. These hormones also encourage the cells to release fat and cholesterol into the bloodstream. Defuse these emotions by practicing stress-management techniques.

- **Review all prescription and over-the-counter drugs with your doctor**. Some medications make your body retain more fluid, further straining your heart. Ask your doctor to assess the medications you're taking for possible adverse side effects.

- **Lower your blood cholesterol, if necessary.** Elevated levels of blood cholesterol increase the risk of atherosclerosis.

- **Keep your blood pressure out of the danger zone.** High blood pressure—a systolic reading above 140 millimeters of mercury (mm HG) and a diastolic reading above 90 mm Hg—is a major risk fac-

UNDERSTANDING CHOLESTEROL

To assess your cardiovascular risk, you need to know your total cholesterol level and the type of cholesterol in your blood. Before the cholesterol can enter the bloodstream it must attach itself to a molecule known as a lipoprotein. (Cholesterol is a fat-like substance, and blood is essentially water; the lipoprotein helps to transport the cholesterol through the blood because fat and water don't mix.)

There are two main types of lipoproteins—low-density lipoproteins (LDLs) and high-density lipoproteins (HDLs). LDLs contribute to the formation of plaque deposits in the arteries and HDLs help to remove those plaque deposits. When a person has high LDL and low HDL levels, the blood often contains high levels of triglycerides (another blood fat) as well. Cardiovascular disease can be caused by either too little HDL or too much LDL.

HOW MUCH IS TOO MUCH?

	Desirable	Borderline	Undesirable
Total cholesterol	below 200	200–239	240+
LDL cholesterol	below 130	130–159	160+
HDL cholesterol	above 45	35–45	below 25

tor for heart attacks. In general, for every one-point reduction in diastolic pressure, your heart attack rate falls by 2 to 3 percent.

- **Know your history**. While there's nothing you can do to control your hereditary predisposition to cardiovascular disease, knowing your medical history can help you manage your risk factors. A family history of early heart attacks, high blood pressure, or stroke greatly increases the risk of developing cardiovascular disease. Anyone whose parent or other close relative has suffered a heart attack or stroke before the age of fifty-five should make a special effort to minimize other risk factors.

WARNING SIGNS

Some people learn that they have heart disease when they experience the chest-crushing pain of angina, and many others don't receive any warning—they simply have their first heart attack.

Heart attack victims often delay seeking medical help, frequently with fatal results. Most heart attack deaths occur in the first two hours, yet studies have found that many people wait four to six hours to get to an emergency room. Never ignore the warning signs of a heart attack. They include:

- Chest pain: an uncomfortable pressure, fullness, squeezing, or crushing feeling in the center of the chest that lasts two minutes or longer

- Severe pain that radiates to the shoulders, neck, arms, jaw, or top of the stomach

- Shortness of breath

- Paleness

- Sweating

- Rapid or irregular pulse

- Dizziness, fainting, or loss of consciousness

Not all of these warning signs occur in every heart attack. And some people, especially older people and diabetics, may not experience symptoms during a heart attack. (These so-called silent heart attacks can be detected only by an electrocardiogram, or EKG.) If you suspect you may be experiencing a heart attack, get emergency medical help immediately. Doctors can prescribe a number of drugs that dissolve clots and reduce oxygen demands on the heart, but these medications are most effective if given within one hour of the onset of a heart attack.

OTHER HERBS USEFUL FOR CARDIOVASCULAR HEALTH

Ginkgo has earned a reputation as a heart-enhancing herb, but other herbs can also help control cardiovascular disease. If you have heart problems or a circulatory disorder, you should be under a doctor's care. As a supplement to your conventional care, these herbs may prove useful (with your doctor's approval, of course):

• *Dandelion (Taraxacum officinale)*: This diuretic herb helps lower blood pressure and relieves chronic liver congestion.

• *Garlic (Allium sativum)*: This herb contains several sulfur compounds that block the biosynthesis of cholesterol. Garlic also helps expand the blood vessel walls, increasing blood flow and lowering blood pressure.

• *Hawthorn (Crataegus oxyacantha)*: This quintessential "heart herb" enhances cardiac output and opens up the peripheral vessels to improve overall circulation.

• *Motherwort (Leonurus cardiaca)*: Small doses of this herb calm heart palpitations and normalize heart function.

61

• *Yarrow (Achillea millefolium)*: This herb acts as a diuretic by dilating peripheral blood vessels. It helps lower blood pressure and reduces pressure on the heart.

FOR MORE INFORMATION

If you experience cardiovascular disease that does not respond to treatment with ginkgo, consider contacting one of the following organizations for additional information:

American Heart Association
7272 Greenville Avenue
Dallas, TX 75231
(214) 373-6300

Citizens for Public Action on Blood Pressure and Cholesterol
P.O. Box 30374
Bethesda, MD 20824
(301) 770-1711

International Atherosclerosis Society
6550 Fannin, No. 1423
Houston, TX 77030
(713) 790-4226

Mended Hearts
7272 Greenville Avenue
Dallas, TX 75231-4966
(214) 706-1442

National Heart, Lung, and Blood Institute
Information Center
National Institutes of Health
(301) 251-1222

National Heart Savers Association
9140 West Dodge Road
Omaha, NE 68114
(402) 398-1993

National Hypertension Association
324 East 30th Street
New York, NY 10016
(212) 889-3557

CHAPTER 5

Ginkgo and Impotence

Sooner or later, it happens to almost every man. Impotence is nothing to feel ashamed of or humiliated about. Still, most men don't like to talk about impotence—a chronic problem in achieving and maintaining an erection long enough to experience intercourse.

While men can remain sexually active into their advanced years, the truth of the matter is that as a normal part of the aging process, the speed of a man's sexual response slows and the intensity of his orgasm declines as testosterone levels drop and the body's circulation grows sluggish. In addition to reducing the need or desire to reach orgasm, these changes can result in the production of a smaller amount of semen during ejaculation. Don't think of these changes—which usually begin to occur in the late forties—as problems. Consider the benefit: You may find that you can enjoy intercourse longer before ejaculation.

And even if you do experience impotence rather than a gradual decline of sexual function, you can rest assured that you are not alone. It is estimated that between 10 and 20 million American men are chronically impotent, including a quarter of men over age sixty-five and more than half of all men over seventy-five. According to the Impotence Resource Center, only 5 percent of those men ever seek treatment, an unfortunate fact since almost 95 percent of impotence cases can be treated successfully.

Thanks to the Food and Drug Administration's recent approval of the oral medication Viagra, the subject of impotence has become less taboo. However, many men who willingly discuss Viagra still feel embarrassed to discuss their personal situation honestly. These feelings are understandable when we consider the well-established social link between sexual potency and manliness; consider that the word "impotence" has its roots in the Latin word *impotentia*, which means "a lack of strength."

Some of the embarrassment could be avoided if men realized that roughly three-fourths of all erection problems have at least some physical cause. To achieve an erection, there must be cooperation among blood vessels, nerves, and tissues; during an erection, the penis becomes engorged with blood as blood vessels enlarge, or dilate, and allow an increased flow. When a man is aroused, the nerves of the penis are stimulated, resulting in an increased blood flow to that organ by 700 percent; this sudden rush of blood expands, strengthens, and hardens the penis into an erection. Since this change is due to nerve stimulation, and since some nerves are controlled in brain centers, a number of drugs that affect the brain can interfere with an erection.

A number of health problems—including diabetes, heart and circulation problems, stroke, epilepsy, Alzheimer's disease, neurological disorders, alcohol and drug abuse, Parkinson's disease, and liver and kidney disease—can cause impotence. So can certain medications, including tranquilizers, diuretics, and antiulcer, antipsychotic, antidepressant, and antihypertensive drugs. Some over-the-counter antihistamines and decongestants can cause temporary impotence.

Other cases of impotence stem from psychological factors, such as relationship problems, stress, anxiety, grief, depression, fatigue, boredom, and guilt. Sexual intimacy can make some people feel very vulnerable, causing a number of stresses and uncomfortable feelings. With patience and treatment, most cases of psychological—as well as physical—impotence can be managed and overcome. Many natural remedies can also help.

PUTTING GINKGO TO THE TEST

Many of the medical problems that respond to ginkgo involve poor blood circulation, and impotence is no exception. Ginkgo improves blood circulation and dilates the veins and arteries without increasing blood pressure, so in many men it can help to overcome impotence. Consider the following studies.

- A 1989 study published in the *Journal of Urology* illustrates ginkgo's effectiveness in the treatment of impotence. The study involved sixty patients who had problems achieving and maintaining erections because of poor circulation in the arteries of the penis. They were given 60 milligrams of ginkgo daily after they failed to respond to treatment with papaverine injections (the drug of choice for most doctors). The participants showed improvement in six to eight weeks. Six months into the twelve- to eighteen-month study, 50 percent of the men were able to sustain erections. About 45 percent of the remaining men noticed some improvement, especially when they were given the ginkgo in conjunction with papaverine; only 5 percent of the study participants showed no improvement at all.

- In another trial, reported in the *Journal of Sex Education and Therapy* in 1991, fifty patients with arterial erectile impotence were given 240 milligrams ginkgo biloba extract for nine months. The men were divided into two groups—twenty had previously benefited from conventional drug treatment for the problem and thirty had not. All of the men who had previously reacted positively to drug treatments regained sexual function in the first three months, and all of those had sufficient erections after six months of treatment. Of the men who had not responded to drug treatment, nineteen out of thirty responded to the ginkgo and eleven others showed some improvement in arterial flow but remained impotent. None of the study participants had any unwanted side effects.

A WORD ABOUT VIAGRA

In 1998 the Food and Drug Administration approved the first oral treatment for impotence. The drug, sildenafil—more commonly known by its brand name, Viagra—is a tablet taken one to two hours before sexual activity to achieve an erection satisfactory for intercourse.

Viagra works by temporarily altering the brain chemistry to relax certain muscles and allow blood flow to the penis. Known side effects appear to be mild and relatively rare; they include stomach upset, nasal congestion, flushing, headaches, and visual disturbances. The drug has only been on the market for a brief time, but there is some anecdotal evidence that suggests its use can cause heart problems in susceptible people.

CONVENTIONAL CARE

When it comes to impotence, a doctor's first task is to rule out a physical cause of the problem. This is usually done by a series of tests to assess the blood flow to the penis, the condition of the spinal cord, and testosterone and blood glucose levels. The doctor may recommend an at-home sleep test to find out if you experience erections during sleep. (If you have no erections during sleep, then there is probably a physical cause for the problem; if you do experience erections at night but not when you are with a partner, the cause is probably psychological.) In addition, your doctor probably will review any drugs you are taking, since impotence is a common side effect of many medications.

If your hormone levels fall below normal, testosterone shots or supplements may be prescribed. If you have inadequate blood flow to the penis, surgery may be required to open or unblock the arteries. And if all else fails, you may want to consider suction-pump devices or penile implants.

OTHER HERBS EFFECTIVE AT TREATING IMPOTENCE

Ginkgo is known to be effective in the treatment of impotence, but two other herbs—ginseng and yohimbe—also have been shown to help with the condition.

• **Ginseng** (*Panax quinquefolius*): This herb has long been considered a mild aphrodisiac. Ginseng may help to reverse impotence by boosting the hormones responsible for sexual response; it also helps with impotence caused by a general lack of vitality and energy. Ginseng helps to strengthen the immune system, decreases fatigue, and serves as an overall tonic. Commercial ginseng products are widely available; follow package directions.

• **Yohimbe** (*Pausinystalia yohimbe*): This herb is the primary ingredient in some prescription drugs used to treat impotence; it works by improving blood flow in the vessels of the penis. It is commercially available, often in so-called male potency formulas. Follow package directions. It should be used only under a doctor's supervision.

FOR MORE INFORMATION

If you experience impotence that does not respond to ginkgo, discuss the matter with your doctor and consider contacting one of the following organizations:

American Association of Sex Educators, Counselors, and Therapists
435 North Michigan Avenue, Suite 1717
Chicago, IL 60611
(312) 644-0828

Impotence Information Center
American Medical Systems
Minneapolis, MN 55440
(800) 543-9632

Impotence Institute of America
10400 Little Patuxent Parkway, Suite 485
Columbia, MD 21044
(410) 715-9605

Potency Restored
8630 Fenton Street, Suite 218
Silver Spring, MD 20910
(301) 588-5777

CHAPTER 6

Ginkgo and Vision and Hearing

Because ginkgo enhances blood circulation
and fights cellular damage caused by free
radicals, it can be very helpful in problems
associated with vision and hearing. Studies
indicate that ginkgo can delay the onset of
certain sensory problems, allowing people
to live without impaired vision or hearing
for a longer time than they would if they did
not take the herb.

VISION

Accurate vision requires healthy eyes, but
sooner or later most people experience
some visual impairment. A person's visual acuity is a measure of visual accu-
racy usually calculated using data from an

eye examination in which the subject reads letters of varying sizes from an eye chart at a distance of twenty feet. Visual acuity is expressed as a fraction of what a person with normal vision would be able to see clearly at twenty feet. In other words, normal vision is 20/20; a person whose visual acuity is 20/40 can see at twenty feet what a healthy person can see at forty feet. In most cases, a person whose visual acuity is 20/60 or worse needs glasses to function well. People with a visual acuity of 20/200 or worse (with glasses) are said to be legally blind.

Vision changes throughout a person's life. The eyes must adjust focus for objects near and far, and this ability changes over the years. For example, most six-year-olds can focus on text as close as two and a half inches; as these children grow older, the lenses of their eyes harden and their ability to focus ultra-close diminishes. In fact, most thirty-year-olds cannot focus clearly unless text is more than six inches away.

While some of these changes are inevitable, ginkgo can help prevent visual impairment, and, in some cases, actually improve eyesight. Ginkgo's ability to fight damage caused by free radicals makes the herb useful in preventing degenerative eye disorders such as macular degeneration and eye damage caused by diabetes.

PROBLEMS WITH FOCUS

Vision problems are often caused by poor blood circulation to the eyes in general and the retina in particular. The sluggish circulation can result in stiff eye muscles and flattened or asymmetrical eyeballs, which can cause nearsightedness (myopia) or farsightedness (hyperopia).

Ginkgo helps improve vision by improving blood circulation in the eyes and by consuming unwanted free radicals. The delicate retina consists of many polyunsaturated fatty acids, which can be damaged easily by free radicals. A number of studies

GETTING TO KNOW YOUR EYES

The eye collects the data for vision, but the act of seeing is actually performed in the brain. The eyes convert light into nerve impulses, which are then sent to the brain. The eye works like a camera, collecting images on the retina in the same way a camera collects images on film.

The eye itself is a sphere consisting of a number of important parts, including the lens, the cornea, the aqueous humor, and the light-sensitive retina. A ring-shaped muscle that surrounds the eye squeezes the lens, changing its shape and focus. The colorful iris opens and shuts to control the amount of light that can enter the eye.

To communicate with the brain, the retina's light-sensitive nerve cells convert the light and images into energy impulses, which are sent to the brain along the optic nerve. There are two basic types of light-converting cells: rods (which work best in low light) and cones (which work best in bright light).

The part of the retina used for acute vision is known as the macula, or macula lutea. This is the part of the eye used to read small print and to focus on tiny details. Many vision problems are caused by macular degeneration, or damage to the macula in the eye.

have confirmed the benefits of using ginkgo in the prevention and treatment of vision problems.

- German researchers examined the retinas of twenty-five people with a median age of seventy-five. The study participants who took 160 milligrams ginkgo per day showed improved vision within four weeks. A second group took 80 milligrams ginkgo daily; their vision did not improve until the dosage was increased to 160 milligrams. Effects were greatest in people with the most damaged tissue; ginkgo had no effect on healthy tissue.

- Animal research conducted in France found that ginkgo can help the retinas withstand oxygen deprivation. The researchers fed rats ginkgo for ten days, then deprived their retinas of oxygen. The ginkgo helped the retinas to withstand damage from oxygen deprivation.

- A 1994 study published in the journal *Ophthalmic Research* looked at the enzymes released by the retina when it is injured or inflamed. The researchers gave eighteen rabbits 40 milligrams of ginkgo daily intravenously; they compared the retinas of these rabbits with the retinas of others that did not receive the herb. They found significantly lower levels of the enzymes indicating damage in the rabbits taking ginkgo.

COLOR BLINDNESS

There are several types of color blindness. In some cases, a person cannot recognize certain colors; other times a person can't differentiate between different shades of the same color. Only rarely does a person see only black and white or, more precisely, shades of gray.

A problem with the retina or optic nerve causes most types of color blindness; typically these problems are inherited and passed from mother to son. (Most females have genes that override the condition.) Other times color blindness is caused by drug or alcohol poisoning. It also can be caused by degenerative damage to the eyes; for example, free-radical damage to the retina can cause people to lose the ability to recognize yellow and blue. A person's ability to appreciate color generally peaks in a the thirties and then declines.

Ginkgo actually can help reverse some types of color blindness, probably due to its diligence as a free-radical scavenger. For example, a French study published in 1988 found that the ability to distinguish colors improved in twenty-nine subjects who took ginkgo for six months.

DIABETES AND VISION

Diabetes is a disease that leaves the body unable to store and use glucose properly. The disease affects the blood vessels, sometimes causing hardening of the arteries, high blood pressure, and other cardiovascular disorders. Often the vessels in the eyes are damaged, which contributes to vision trouble.

Ginkgo can help the body protect the retinas. In a 1986 study, French researchers investigated the impact of ginkgo on the retinas of diabetic rats. Diabetes is known to damage the retinas by causing capillaries in the retinas to thicken. The researchers found that the condition of rats' retinas improved when they were given ginkgo. Rats given ginkgo before they developed diabetes actually resisted some damage to the retinas caused by the disease. Unfortunately, no studies have been completed on the impact of ginkgo on the vision of humans with diabetes, but it would be prudent for humans to use the herb rather than wait for clinical proof, since the herb is harmless at the recommended doses.

MACULAR DEGENERATION

Macular degeneration is one of the leading causes of blindness in Americans over age sixty-five. It involves gradual damage to the macula, the part of the retina used for seeing the center of a visual field. The problem is caused by a buildup of a lipid-containing, brownish pigment known as lipofuscin, which is produced by the degeneration of cells.

During the early phases of macular degeneration, the blood vessels behind the retinas break down and begin to leak fluid. Scar tissue forms, creating a blockage in the middle of the macula that creates a blind spot in the center of vision. As the condition worsens, the blind spot grows larger.

A number of studies have shown that

ginkgo can help prevent or slow the progression of macular degeneration. Ginkgo is widely used in Europe as a treatment for the condition. Consider the evidence.

- In 1986 French researchers conducted a study of ten people with macular degeneration; half received ginkgo and half a placebo. The ginkgo group experienced an improvement in long-distance vision. Despite the small sample size, the results were considered statistically significant.

- In the *Journal of the Advancement of Medicine* in 1993, two researchers reviewed the literature concerning specific nutrients that have proven effective in the treatment of macular degeneration and cataracts. The nutrients found to help with these vision problems include ginkgo, as well as zinc, taurine, vitamin A, vitamin B2, vitamin C, vitamin E, selenium, beta-carotene, and flavonoids.

AN OUNCE OF PREVENTION

To minimize your risk of developing vision problems, protect your eyes from ultraviolet light by avoiding direct sunlight and by wearing dark sunglasses and a wide-brim hat when outdoors. Since free radicals appear to be the leading cause of cataracts associated with aging, eating a diet rich in antioxidants can help protect the eyes.

Of course, regular eye exams are necessary to detect and treat cataracts in their early stages. Have your eyes tested by an ophthalmologist at least every five years. An ophthalmologist is a medical doctor specializing in diseases and surgery of the eye; an optometrist assesses the need for glasses and writes prescriptions for glasses or contact lenses; an optician fills prescriptions for eyeglasses or contact lenses.

For a referral to an ophthalmologist in your area, check the Yellow Pages or call the American Academy of Ophthalmology at (415) 561-8500.

HEARING

About 8.5 million Americans have trouble hearing, and about 300,000 of these people are either completely or nearly deaf. The majority of these people are adults whose hearing problems can be attributed at least partially to the cumulative effect of a lifetime of noise. That should come as no surprise when you consider that the human ear is a remarkably delicate organ. Sound waves enter the ear, causing minute vibrations on the eardrum. These vibrations stimulate the movement of tiny hairs in the inner ear; the hairs in turn convert these movements into nerve impulses, which are then transmitted to the brain by the auditory nerve. Then at last the brain receives the signal and registers sound. As we age, the tiny hairs deteriorate and don't conduct sound vibrations as well as they once did, causing hearing loss.

Age-related hearing loss (known as *presbycusis*, from the Greek work meaning "old hearing") often begins in the twenties, but the changes are so subtle that they usually go unnoticed until age sixty or so, when loss of middle- and low-frequency hearing makes it difficult to discern speech. Fully 60 percent of people over age sixty-five and 90 percent of those over age seventy-five have some hearing loss.

In addition to damage to the hairs, age can affect other structures in the ear. For example, the bones in the ear can become stiff and less responsive to vibration, and the eardrum itself may become thicker and less flexible. Some people inherit a tendency for the bones in the ear to overgrow, causing other types of problems.

Hearing also can be compromised by other health problems, such as heart disease, high blood pressure, diabetes, and other circulatory disorders that can diminish the blood supply to the ears, causing damage. Acute ear infections can damage the ear structure, leading to permanent hearing loss.

There are three types of hearing loss: conductive, sensorineural, and central deafness.

- **Conductive hearing loss** is caused by a blockage in the inner ear, usually earwax packed into the ear canal. Infection, fluid in the inner ear, and abnormal bone growth also can cause this type of hearing loss. Symptoms include voices sounding muffled while your own voice sounds loud; it may be accompanied by tinnitus, or ringing, hissing, buzzing, or clicking sounds in the ears.

- **Sensorineural hearing loss** is caused by problems with the acoustic nerve in the inner ear. In most cases people with this type of damage have trouble understanding speech but remain sensitive to loud sounds; they also may experience tinnitus. Sensorineural hearing loss can be the result of aging, exposure to loud noises, or a reaction to certain medications, such as aspirin, some antibiotics, and antihypertensive drugs. An exceptionally loud noise (such as an explosion) can destroy the hairs outright. At somewhat lower levels (a rock concert or a car stereo at full blast, for example), the damage can be slow and steady.

- **Central deafness** is a rare condition caused by damage to the hearing centers of the brain. The person can hear normally but cannot understand what is heard. This condition can be caused by stroke, prolonged high fever, or a blow to the head.

While it can be difficult to prevent some of these problems, ginkgo appears able to prevent or reverse some of the damage. Consider the evidence.

- In a 1986 study French researchers found that ginkgo can help in the treatment of cochlear deafness (hearing loss caused by damage to the cochlea, the structure that transforms the vibrations of sound into nerve impulses sent to the brain). They concluded that ginkgo worked by improving blood circulation in the ears. Half the study participants were given 320 milligrams ginkgo daily, and the other participants were given a type of drug called an alpha-blocker. While all of the subjects experienced some improvement, 52 percent of those taking ginkgo extract showed substantial hearing improvement, compared to 35 percent of those in the group that took the alpha-blocker.

- In another study, researchers compared the effectiveness of 80 milligrams ginkgo and alpha-blockers in the treatment of patients who became deaf suddenly, either due to a sudden loud noise or a sudden drop in air pressure. Ten people received the ginkgo, and ten were given the alpha-blockers. Among the drug group, three had very good results, three had fair results, and four did not improve. Among the ginkgo group, seven people had excellent results, one had a fair result, and one did not improve. The hearing was most improved on the tenth day of treatment.

TINNITUS (RINGING IN THE EARS)

While hearing loss is a problem, so is never being able to experience silence. About 36 million Americans suffer from tinnitus, a periodic or unrelenting noise—ringing, buzzing, roaring, hissing, and whistling sounds—in the ears. The acoustic nerve in the ear responds to stimulation. People with tinnitus can experience symptoms often caused by poor blood circulation.

Ginkgo helps ease tinnitus by improving blood circulation and improving nutrient transport to the nerves of the inner ear. Consider the evidence.

- In 1986 French researchers examined the impact of ginkgo on tinnitus. The three-month, double-blind study involved 103 patients who had had tinnitus for less than one year. One group was given 320 milligrams ginkgo daily for thirty days; the others were given a placebo. All of the people receiving the ginkgo improved much more than those taking the placebo. Another study showed similar improvement among people taking 60 to 160 milligrams ginkgo daily.

- In a 1979 study, researchers found ginkgo successful in treating people with tinnitus, vertigo, or hearing loss. The hearing problems were associated with various vascular disorders, trauma, or infection. Half the study participants were given 120 milligrams ginkgo per day; the other half received 15 milligrams nicergoline per day, a drug used to treat the problems in Europe. The ginkgo was particularly effective in treating vertigo. While nicergoline also worked, the ginkgo was considered superior.

- A three-month study examined the impact of ginkgo in forty-two patients with tinnitus or another hearing problem. The dosage of ginkgo varied between 120 and 160 milligrams, depending on the extent of the problem. The results were good or very good in 40 percent of the people taking the ginkgo, and only 21 percent did not experience improvement in their condition. Among the people with tinnitus, the success rate was 82 percent, with 53 percent experiencing a complete remission of symptoms.

- In another study done in 1979, fully 70 percent of the study participants with vertigo and hearing loss improved with ginkgo biloba extract. Ginkgo was least effective in people who had hearing problems for an extended period of time. Of the twenty-six people with vertigo who participated in the study, twenty-four were satisfied with their improvement using ginkgo.

VERTIGO AND DIZZINESS

Dizziness or vertigo (the feeling of falling) can be caused by a disruption within the inner ear, which is sometimes caused by something as simple as an inner ear infection or the common cold, or as complex as circulation problems caused by atherosclerosis.

At other times, dizziness and vertigo are caused by Ménière's disease, named for the French physician Prosper Ménière, who first described the condition in 1861. Ménière's disease is a disorder of the inner ear that causes vertigo, tinnitus, a feeling of pressure in the ear, and fluctuating hearing loss. The condition usually comes on as attacks that last two to four hours.

Ginkgo has been found to be effective in the treatment of dizziness and vertigo. Consider the evidence:

- In a three-month, multi-center study reported in the French journal *La Presse Medicale* in 1986, researchers tested sixty-seven people who had recently developed balance problems. Thirty-four were given 160 milligrams of ginkgo daily and the others received a placebo. After ninety days, 75 percent of the people taking ginkgo had improved, compared to just 18 percent of the people taking the placebo.

ANOTHER OUNCE OF PREVENTION

The best way to protect your hearing is to avoid bombarding your ears with loud noises, which can cause permanent damage to the middle ear. Noises of 85 to 90 decibels or higher are considered damaging. This level is lower than most people realize. (Normal speech is usually 65 to 70 decibels.) If you listen to loud music, work around loud machinery, or use many everyday appliances, such as vacuum cleaners and lawn mowers, you may be exposed to excessive noise. So-called impulse noises, such as explosions from firearms or firecrackers, are particularly dangerous because they are so sudden. If you are going to be exposed to loud noises, wear protective earplugs, which are sold in drugstores and sports goods stores.

You also can prevent hearing loss by taking care of ear infections promptly. Left untreated, an infection of the middle ear can cause permanent hearing loss. Ear infections usually can be cleared up with a ten-day course of antibiotics.

You also can avoid some hearing problems by getting your hearing checked regularly. Between the ages of fifty and sixty-four, have a hearing exam at least once every five years. After age sixty-five, have your primary care physician test your hearing as part of your regular annual physical exam.

A simple but crude test to measure high-frequency hearing loss is to rub your thumb and forefinger together near your ear. If you can't hear the rubbing sound, your hearing may be impaired.

Be on the lookout for signs of hearing damage. Contact your doctor if you recognize any of these signs in yourself:

- You hear better some days than others.
- You fail to hear words or phrases in conversation.
- You find it difficult to conduct a conversation in a large group.
- You often accuse other people of mumbling or not speaking clearly.
- You experience dizziness or a loss of balance.
- You hear noises in your head.

These can all be signs of a hearing problem that should be treated by a physician.

FOR MORE INFORMATION

If you experience vision or hearing problems, discuss the matter with your doctor, then try using ginkgo to help manage the symptoms. You may also want to contact one or more of the following organizations:

ON VISION

American Academy of Ophthalmology
655 Beach Street
San Francisco, CA 94109
(415) 561-8500

American Foundation for Vision Awareness
243 North Lindbergh Boulevard
St. Louis, MO 63141
(800) 927-2382

American Optometric Association
1505 Prince Street, Suite 300
Alexandria, VA 22314
(703) 739-9200

National Eye Institute
Building 31, Room 6-A32
31 Center Drive
MSC-2510
Bethesda, MD 20892-2510
(301) 496-5248

To find out if your ophthalmologist is board
certified, contact:

American Board of Ophthalmology
111 Presidential Boulevard
Suite 241
Bala Cynwyd, PA 19004
(610) 664-1175

ON HEARING

**American Speech-Language-Hearing
Association**
10801 Rockville Pike
Rockville, MD 20852
(301) 897-5700; (301) 897-8682;
(800) 638-8255

Better Hearing Institute
5021-B Backlick Road
Annandale, VA 22003
(800) EAR-WELL

International Hearing Society
20361 Middlebelt Road
Livonia, MI 48152
(810) 478-2610

National Information Center on Deafness
Gallaudet University
Health Department
800 Florida Avenue, N.E.
Washington, DC 20002

National Institute on Deafness and Other Communication Disorders Clearinghouse
1 Communication Avenue
Bethesda, MD 20892-3456
(800) 241-1044
(800) 241-1055 (TDD)

SHHH (Self Help for Hard of Hearing People, Inc.)
7910 Woodmont Avenue, Suite 1200
Bethesda, MD 20814
(301) 657-2248
(301) 657-2249 (TDD)

For free information on hearing or a free over-the-phone hearing test, call:

(800) 222-EARS
(800) 345-EARS (in Pennsylvania)

GOOD FOR THE SENSE OF SMELL TOO

In addition to improving vision and hearing, ginkgo also appears to help people who have an impaired ability to smell. More than 200,000 people visit their doctor each year because they cannot smell properly or because their sense of smell is overly heightened. Many of these smell disorders occur in people with Alzheimer's disease or Parkinson's disease; both conditions are caused by problems with brain biochemistry. Effective dosages vary depending on the severity of the problem and the overall health of the person taking the ginkgo.

CHAPTER 7

Other Uses of Ginkgo

Many of ginkgo's healing effects are a result of the herb's ability to support and strengthen the circulatory system. A healthy circulatory system is essential for good health. Ginkgo also helps with a number of health problems because it blocks a compound known as platelet-activating factor, or PAF. The PAF activates the immune system, in particular triggering inflammation and blood clotting. When the PAF excites the immune system too much, it can trigger allergies, asthma, and other immune-system responses. For reasons that are not fully understood, ginkgo helps to protect against these exaggerated PAF responses, which in turn helps control the immune response.

This chapter summarizes some of the

conditions that researchers have shown respond well to the use of ginkgo.

ALLERGIES

It starts out with a simple sneeze. Then one sneeze turns into three, then five, then the eyes begin to water and itch. These aren't the symptoms of the common cold but rather of allergies.

An allergy is the body's exaggerated response to an irritant that is breathed (such as dust mites, pollen, mold, or pet dander), eaten (such as dairy products, wheat, or peanuts), or touched (such as wool, fabric softener, or perfume). Inside the body, this perceived invader, or allergen, is attacked by IgE antibodies (immunoglobulin E). The antibodies set off a chain reaction that leads to any number of symptoms, including runny nose and inflammation of the nasal passages, hives, eczema, arthritis, itching, diarrhea, and headaches. Most people aren't bothered by allergies because their antibodies respond moderately to the foreign substances. The immune systems of people with allergies, however, overreact to these symptoms, creating the allergic response.

If your allergies bother you, you may want to be tested to find out exactly which allergen is causing the problem. Once you know what you're up against, you can try to avoid contact with the substances that bother you. In addition, you can use ginkgo to minimize the allergic response. Researchers believe that the terpene molecules in ginkgo (also known as the ginkgolides) interfere with the platelet-activating factor, which is one of the major chemical mediators in asthma, inflammation, and allergies. The ginkgolides inhibit the PAF on a cellular level, minimizing allergic and asthmatic responses. Several studies have backed up this finding.

- In 1990 researchers examined the role of ginkgo on PAF production in twelve people with allergies. The PAF levels were measured in the study participants before and after they were given 120 milligrams ginkgo extract daily. Without the ginkgo, the participants showed an immediate and acute reaction when exposed to an allergen; when they were given the herb, they were better able to tolerate the allergen.

- A 1988 study published in *The Lancet* reported that people taking 240 milligrams ginkgo extract daily for three weeks experienced a dramatic improvement in a condition known as systemic mastocytosis. This condition involves the abnormal proliferation of mast cells in some tissues, which results in redness of the face and trunk and recurrent facial flushing, conjunctivitis, palpitations, dizziness, abdominal pain, diarrhea, nausea, and severe low blood pressure.

Do Away With Allergens

The best way to deal with allergies is to avoid exposing yourself to the substances that trigger outbreaks. Keeping your house scrupulously clean may help prevent some allergic reactions. Cover the mattresses with plastic; remove the carpet in the bedroom, and vacuum all rugs frequently. Keep your house, especially your bedroom, as clean and dust-free as possible.

Vacuum cleaners with special dust-trapping filters may prove helpful. For more information on vacuums and other products for allergy sufferers, contact:

Allergy Control Products
96 Danbury Road
Ridgefield, CT 06877
(800) 422-DUST

National Allergy Supply
P.O. Box 1658
440 Georgia Highway 120
Duluth, GA 30136
(800) 522-1448

FOR MORE INFORMATION

If you have a problem with allergies that
does not respond to treatment with ginkgo,
consider contacting one or more of the following organizations:

**American Academy of Environmental
Medicine**
P.O. Box 16106
Denver, CO 80216
(303) 622-9755

**Asthma and Allergy Foundation of
America**
1124 15th Street, NW
Washington, DC 20005
(202) 466-7643
(800) 7-ASTHMA

ASTHMA

In most cases, asthma develops in childhood. Asthma is a lung disease in which the bronchial tubes narrow, swell, and become clogged with mucus, often in response to an allergen. During an attack, the asthmatic person strains to inhale and exhale; this straining creates a wheezing or whistling sound. Often the asthmatic person coughs uncontrollably and experiences a tightness in the chest and a shortness of breath during an attack. Asthma has become more common—and more serious—recently; the number of asthma-related deaths has increased by 40 percent between 1982 and 1995. No one knows the reason for this increase, but experts believe it is caused by an increase in exposure to indoor allergens, and poor overall air quality.

Most people with asthma are allergic to one or more irritants. The most common allergens for asthmatic people are dust and mold, animal dander, dairy products, pollen, and a variety of drugs, especially those related to penicillin and other antibiotics.

Ginkgo is helpful in the treatment of asthma and chronic bronchitis. In fact, the ginkgolides in the herb inhibit bronchoconstriction by blocking the PAF. A number of studies have shown that ginkgo can be an important part of an approach to controlling asthma attacks.

- For example, a study published in 1987 in the journal *Prostaglandins* reported that the ginkgolides found in ginkgo inhibit bronchial constriction in asthmatic patients for up to six hours after they were exposed to an allergen known to cause an asthmatic response.

- In a 1987 study, people diagnosed with asthma were given either 120 milligrams ginkgo biloba extract or a placebo. After three days of treatment, the participants were exposed to allergenic dust mites or pollens. The people taking the ginkgo experienced much less bronchoconstriction for up to six hours after the exposure. None of the study participants reported any unwanted side effects.

- In 1992 the journal *Drugs & Aging* reported a study of seventeen asthmatics who were treated with ginkgo biloba extract for one year. People who were given the ginkgo improved in their ability to manage the disease.

- Another study used isolated ginkgo-lides—ginkgolides A, B, and C, also known as BN 52063—to assess the impact of ginkgo on asthma. These ginkgo-lides were known to antagonize the platelet-activating factors and block bronchoconstriction caused by either exercise or exposure to an allergen.

FOR MORE INFORMATION

If you have a problem with asthma that does not respond to treatment with ginkgo, consider contacting one of the following organizations for additional information:

Asthma and Allergy Foundation of America
1125 15th Street, N.W.
Suite 502
Washington, DC 20005
(202) 466-7643

Joint Council of Allergy, Asthma, and Immunology
50 N. Brockway
No. 3-3
Palatine, IL 60667
(847) 934-1918

DEPRESSION

At some point in their lives, most people experience depression. For reasons we don't fully understand depression occurs significantly more often in women than men. Depression isn't the same thing as sadness—we all feel sad in response to certain situations. Depression, however, involves ongoing, unrelenting feelings of worthlessness and pessimism. In mild depression, these feelings may linger for weeks; in severe cases, they can become completely incapacitating.

Depression can be caused by the chemistry of the brain. Other times the illness is triggered by physical conditions, such as stroke, hepatitis, chronic fatigue syndrome, chronic stress, thyroid disease, menopause, alcoholism, seasonal affective disorder, or drug abuse. In some cases, over-the-counter antihistamines and other drugs can cause depression.

Ginkgo has been shown to be effective in the treatment of some cases of depression, probably because it increases the amount of oxygen available to the brain. The added oxygen and other nutrients may help the depressed brain adjust its biochemistry and reverse the depression in much the same way that exercise has been shown to relieve depression.

Some researchers recommend the use of ginkgo in combination with prescription antidepressant drugs, such as tricyclics and tetracyclics. If you are taking any medications for the treatment of depression, do not begin taking ginkgo or any other drug without discussing the matter with your doctor first.

WARNING SIGNS OF DEPRESSION

Although it can be difficult to tell the difference between clinical depression and common sadness, there are certain warning signs. These signs include:

- Changes in sleep—either insomnia or excessive sleepiness
- Changes in weight and eating habits—either weight gain or weight loss
- Loss of sexual desire or libido
- Chronic fatigue or tiredness
- Low self-esteem or self-worth
- Loss of productivity at work, home, or school
- Inability to concentrate or think clearly
- Withdrawal or isolation
- Loss of interest in activities that were once enjoyable
- Anger or irritability
- Trouble accepting praise or affirmations
- Feeling slow, that every activity takes a supreme effort
- Apprehensive about the future

- Frequent weeping or sobbing
- Thoughts of suicide or death

These are all warning signs and diagnostic criteria for depression. If you or a loved one experiences three or more of these symptoms for two weeks or longer, contact a doctor or mental health professional for help. Don't try to treat serious depression by yourself. And if you or someone you're concerned about feels suicidal, immediately seek help from a specialist or a twenty-four-hour hot line; look in the phone book under "Suicide Prevention."

FOR MORE INFORMATION

If you experience symptoms of depression that do not respond to treatment with ginkgo, consider requesting additional information from your doctor or from one or more of the following organizations:

Depressives Anonymous: Recovering from Depression
329 East 62nd Street
New York, NY 10021
(212) 689-2600

Depression Awareness, Recognition, and Treatment (D/ART)
National Institute of Mental Health
9000 Rockville Pike
Bethesda, MD 20892
(800) 421-4211

Depression and Related Affective Disorders Association
Johns Hopkins Hospital
600 North Wolfe Street

Baltimore, MD 21287
(410) 955-4647

**Foundation for Depression and Manic
Depression**
24 East 81st Street, Suite 2B
New York, NY 10028
(212) 772-3400

**National Depressive and Manic
Depressive Association**
730 North Franklin Street, Suite 501
Chicago, IL 60610
(800) 826-3632
(312) 642-0049

**National Foundation for Depressive
Illness**
P.O. Box 2257
New York, NY 10116
(212) 268-4260

National Mental Health Association
1021 Prince Street
Alexandria, VA 22314
(800) 243-2525
(703) 684-7722

DIABETES

People with diabetes must carefully monitor their blood-sugar levels. If the levels rise too high and stay there too long, they can damage the nerves and blood vessels, which can cause a number of additional health problems, including blindness, infection, kidney problems, stroke, and heart disease. On the other hand, if blood-sugar levels drop too low—even for a few minutes—a diabetic person can become confused and lose consciousness.

In healthy people, the pancreas balances the sugar levels in the bloodstream. But for the fourteen million Americans with diabetes mellitus, the pancreas cannot properly convert food into energy, either because the body does not produce enough insulin (a hormone produced in the pancreas to regulate blood-sugar levels) or because the body doesn't properly use the insulin it does produce. Diabetic people must monitor their blood-sugar levels, making adjustments in their diet and exercise levels or their medications and insulin injections to meet changing conditions.

There are two basic types of diabetes: the more severe form, known as Type I, insulin-dependent, or juvenile diabetes (about 15 percent of cases); and Type II, noninsulin-dependent, or adult-onset diabetes (about 85 percent of cases).

- Type I diabetes usually strikes sometime between the onset of puberty and age thirty. It is caused by damage to the insulin-producing cells in the pancreas. For some reason it affects males more often than females.

- Type II diabetes usually occurs in middle-age and older people, especially those who are overweight. In most cases losing as little as ten or fifteen pounds helps control Type II diabetes. In this type of diabetes, the pancreas produces insulin, but the sugar remains in the bloodstream. This more subtle version of the disease often goes undetected until complications arise. Ultimately, up to 60 percent of Type II diabetics need supplemental insulin if they do not lose weight and exercise regularly.

Both Type I and Type II diabetes seem to have a genetic component as well. Other possible causes include an immune response following a viral infection that destroys the cells in the pancreas. Diabetes can also occur in the wake of other diseases, such as thyroid disorders, inflammation of the pancreas, or problems with the pituitary gland. In addition, about 5 percent of women develop diabetes during pregnancy (gestational diabetes), although the symptoms usually disappear after the baby is born.

While not all cases of diabetes can be prevented, many can. People should maintain a healthy weight (most diabetics weight thirty to sixty pounds more than they should); eat a low-fat, high-fiber diet; and exercise regularly. Studies have shown that vigorous exercise can lower the risk of developing Type II diabetes by one-third. Many experts consider exercise the most effective way to prevent noninsulin-dependent diabetes.

Ginkgo also has been shown to help deal with some of the complications of diabetes, specifically damage to the retinas and to the nerves. Consider these studies and discuss with your physician whether ginkgo is right for you:

- In 1986 researchers measured the effect of ginkgo on eye damage caused by diabetes in rats. The researchers injected the rats with a drug that would produce diabetes. Thereafter, some of the test animals received ginkgo, and the others did not. After two months of treatment, the rats that received the ginkgo had superior retinal functioning compared to the rats that did not receive the herb. This study suggests that ginkgo can help protect the eyes against diabetic retinopathy.

- A 1992 study involving humans also concluded that ginkgo can be helpful in treating people with diabetic neuropathy, especially when combined with the B vitamin folic acid. Study participants who received 100 milligrams ginkgo extract and 15 milligrams folic acid daily for fourteen days experienced significant improvement in nerve conductivity compared with the participants who received a placebo with or without the vitamin.

- Another study involved ten people with nerve damage caused by diabetes, lead poisoning, excessive protein in the blood, or peripheral vascular disease. The participants received intravenous doses of 87.5 milligrams ginkgo extract daily. After two weeks, seven of the ten participants reported improved sensation in the affected area.

FOR MORE INFORMATION

If you experience symptoms of diabetes, inform your doctor immediately. Discuss the use of ginkgo in your overall strategy to manage the disease. You may also want to contact one or more of the following groups for more information:

American Diabetes Association
National Center
P.O. Box 25757
1660 Duke Street
Alexandria, VA 22314
(703) 549-1500

Diabetes Research Institute Foundation
3440 Hollywood Boulevard, Suite 100
Hollywood, FL 33021
(305) 964-4040

International Diabetes Center
3800 Park Nicollet Boulevard
Minneapolis, MN 55416
(612) 927-3393

Joslin Diabetes Center
One Joslin Place
Boston, MA 02215
(617) 732-2415

HEMORRHOIDS

Most people don't like to talk about them, but four out of five Americans experience hemorrhoids at some point in their lives. Hemorrhoids, those inflamed and widened veins that look like purple skin, grow around the anus and can be painful and itchy. While they affect people of all ages, about half of people over age fifty experience hemorrhoids at any given time.

Hemorrhoids (sometimes called piles) can appear either outside or inside the anus. They can be caused by constipation, obesity, pregnancy, improper diet, lack of exercise, heavy lifting, prolonged periods of sitting, or liver damage. The condition tends to run in families, either because people inherit delicate veins or because they acquire similar lifestyle and personal habits that can exacerbate the problem. Either way, many cases of hemorrhoids can be prevented by carefully monitoring bowel function.

Ginkgo helps improve blood circulation in the lower extremities, making it useful in the treatment of hemorrhoids. Consider the following.

- A 1971 study of thirty-six people with advanced hemorrhoids reported good to very good results in 86 percent of the patients who were treated with ginkgo biloba extract.

- A 1974 study of twenty people with hemorrhoidal inflammation and anal fissures found that ginkgo biloba extract is very effective in treating the pain associated with rectal bleeding caused by hemorrhoidal inflammation. The herb was less effective at healing the rectal fissures.

PREVENTING HEMORRHOIDS

While some people tend to be more susceptible to hemorrhoids than others, you can avoid many episodes by not straining or pushing during bowel movements. In many cases you also can prevent hemorrhoids by drinking at least eight 8-ounce glasses of water a day and eating a high-fiber diet rich in fresh fruits and vegetables.

If you develop hemorrhoids, you will experience rectal pain and tenderness, itching, and sometimes bleeding. Often the first sign is bright-red blood in the stool, caused by the pressure of a bowel movement. The bleeding is usually minor. Dark, tarry blood in the stool could indicate a more severe internal bleeding problem and should be brought to a doctor's attention as soon as possible.

FOR MORE INFORMATION

If you have a problem with hemorrhoids that does not respond to treatment with ginkgo, consider contacting one of the following organizations for additional information:

American Gastroenterological Association
7910 Woodmont Avenue
Suite 700
Bethesda, MD 20814
(301) 654-2055

Digestive Diseases National Coalition
507 Capital Court, N.E.
Suite 200
Washington, DC 20005
(202) 544-7497

National Digestive Diseases Information Clearinghouse
2 Information Way
Bethesda, MD 20892-3570
(301) 654-3810

MIGRAINE HEADACHE

When your head hurts, everything hurts. While there are a number of different causes of headaches, there are two main types: tension and migraine headaches. Tension headaches are characterized by a steady, dull pain starting at the front or back of the head, then spreading over the entire head. Migraine headaches, on the other hand, involve a throbbing, piercing, intense pain.

Migraine headaches begin to throb when the blood vessels in the head expand more than normal, often in response to food allergies, hormonal changes, stress, and other factors. Migraine pain can last for hours or even days and may be accompanied by nausea and vomiting. Migraines are surprisingly common.

Because ginkgo helps to dilate the vessels and promote proper cerebral circulation, it may be effective in some cases of migraine headache. Migraines are believed to be the cause of a malfunction in vasodilation and constriction of blood vessels in the brain. By heightening blood flow and oxygenation of brain tissue, many headaches can be prevented.

Headaches can be caused by emotional stress, infectious disease, teeth and mouth disorders, eye problems, cold, sinusitis, anemia, gastrointestinal disorders, very high blood pressure, head injury, gas poisoning, and sensitivity to monosodium glutamate, among others.

- Ginkgo appears very effective at treating migraine headaches. In a 1975 study, ginkgo biloba extract was given to people suffering from migraine headaches. Eighty percent experienced either a significant remission or a reduction in symptoms.

- A double-blind study reported similar findings in people who had suffered from migraines for a considerable period of time. The researchers concluded that ginkgo could be used as an effective treatment for migraine.

FOR MORE INFORMATION

If you have a problem with migraine headaches that does not respond to treatment with ginkgo, discuss the matter with your doctor and consider contacting one of the following organizations for additional information:

American Association for the Study of Headache
19 Mantua Road
Mount Royal, NJ 08061
(609) 423-0043

National Headache Foundation
428 W. Saint James Place
2nd Floor
Chicago, IL 60614
(773) 388-6399

MULTIPLE SCLEROSIS

Multiple sclerosis (MS) is a disease characterized by damage to the linings of the nerve membranes.

As noted in the discussion of allergies and asthma, ginkgo contains ginkgolides that interfere with platelet-activating factors; PAF plays an important role in multiple sclerosis, just as it does in allergies and asthma. Consider the evidence and discuss with your physician whether ginkgo is right for you.

- A 1992 study examined the impact of intravenous ginkgo on the course of multiple sclerosis. For the study, ten participants whose MS was in acute relapse were given a five-day course of ginkgolide B intravenously. Eight participants experienced improvement in their neurological performance just two days after treatment began. The improvement extended six days after the treatment ended.

FOR MORE INFORMATION

If you have multiple sclerosis you need to be under a doctor's care. Discuss with your doctor the use of ginkgo as part of your overall treatment. For more information on the disease, consider contacting one of the following organizations:

Multiple Sclerosis Association of America
706 Haddonfield Road
Cherry Hill, NJ 08002-2652
(609) 488-4500

Multiple Sclerosis Foundation
6350 N. Andrews Avenue
Ft. Lauderdale, FL 33309-2130
(954) 776-6805

PMS—PREMENSTRUAL SYNDROME

According to the Premenstrual Institute, up to 40 percent of women of childbearing age suffer from premenstrual syndrome (PMS) to some degree. Some women develop symptoms in puberty, while others don't suffer the effects of PMS until after giving birth or experiencing a significant emotional stress.

Premenstrual syndrome involves a number of unpleasant physical and emotional side effects, including the following:

- Acne
- Aggression
- Anger
- Anxiety
- Bloating or water retention
- Depression

- Dizziness

- Food cravings

- Headaches

- Inability to concentrate

- Short temper

- Swollen hands and feet

- Tender breasts

Typically, the symptoms begin to appear during the week before a woman's menstrual cycle or during ovulation, and they do not subside until after the beginning of menstruation. PMS symptoms sometimes are present during the week after a woman finishes menstruation.

Some women can control the symptoms by avoiding certain foods (such as caffeine and sugar), by getting more rest and exercise (especially aerobic exercise), or by taking anti-inflammatory medications. Ginkgo may help to ease the symptoms of PMS. Consider the following.

- One study involved 165 women between the ages of eighteen and forty-five who suffered from severe PMS. The participants were given ginkgo extract from the sixteenth day of the menstrual cycle to the fifth day of the next cycle. Ginkgo was found to be effective against various symptoms of PMS, particularly breast changes. It was also found to be helpful with the mood changes and emotional symptoms associated with PMS.

For More Information

If you experience symptoms of premenstrual syndrome that do not respond to treatment with ginkgo, discuss the matter with your doctor and consider contacting one of the following organizations for additional information:

American Gynecological and Obstetrical Society
University of Utah
50 North Medical Drive
Salt Lake City, UT 84132
(801) 581-5501

National Center for Education in Maternal and Child Health
2000 15th Street, N.
Suite 701
Arlington, VA 22201-2617
(703) 524-7802

National Maternal and Child Health Clearinghouse
2070 Chain Bridge Road

Suite 450
Vienna, VA 22182-2536
(703) 356-1964

Society for Menstrual Cycle Research
10559 N. 104th Place
Scottsdale, AZ 85258
(602) 451-9731

SKIN DAMAGE

Excessive exposure to the sun can cause skin cancer and accelerate aging of the skin. Researchers believe that the ultraviolet B radiation in sunlight damages the light-sensitive proteins in the skin. The ultraviolet A rays trigger the production of additional melanin (the tanning agent) to shield the body from the sun's rays. Eventually, the tan fades and the cells with melanin slough off, causing a loss of cells. The skin then loses its elasticity and begins to sag.

Ginkgo helps to minimize damage caused by the sun. It gobbles up the damaging free radicals and strengthens the capillaries, which help to heal the skin. Consider the evidence.

- In 1992 researchers found that ginkgo, taken in combination with vitamin A, vi-

tamin E, and selenium, helped to minimize cell damage caused by sunlight.

- Researchers reported in 1992 that ginkgo
  helped minimize free-radical damage to
  organ tissues that had been exposed to
  ultraviolet radiation.

FOR MORE INFORMATION

If you would like additional information about your skin, discuss the matter with your doctor and consider contacting one of the following organizations for additional information:

American Skin Association
150 East 58th Street
33rd Floor
New York, NY 10155-0002
(212) 753-8260

American Academy of Dermatology
930 N. Meacham Road
Schaumburg, IL 60173
(847) 330-0230

Dermatology Foundation
1560 Sherman Avenue
Suite 870
Evanston, IL 60201-4802
(708) 328-2256

Now that you have an appreciation for the many healing benefits of ginkgo, you are ready to learn how to use this herb as part of your daily health routine. The following section, "Using Ginkgo," will describe how to buy and use this plant to improve your overall health.

PART THREE

Using Ginkgo

CHAPTER 8

How to Buy and Use Ginkgo

Ginko is one of the most popular herbs on the market today. It is easy to find in the herb section of drugstores and health food stores; it is also available by mail order and on the Internet. Finding ginkgo won't be a problem; choosing the product that is right for you is a bigger challenge.

Ginkgo is available as dried leaves, powdered or liquid extracts, teas, and homeopathic preparations, among other forms. Some people use fresh ginkgo leaves, but others who don't have access to the leaves or who don't want to prepare a product from scratch may prefer to use commercial products. Commercially prepared herbs offer an easy, inexpensive, and effective way to take ginkgo.

Most herbal manufacturers standardize

extracts of ginkgo leaves and use them to form tablets, liquids, and intravenous preparations (which are not used in the United States). The German phytomedicine company Schwabe has been producing ginkgo extracts for more than twenty years, based on a process developed by Dr. Willmar Schwabe. His twenty-seven-step process takes two weeks, using the leaves of the ginkgo tree that have been harvested in late summer or early fall (when their active ingredients peak in concentration). The active ingredients are isolated and standardized during the extraction, so that the strength is consistent from dose to dose. It takes about fifty pounds of leaves to yield one pound of extract, which is then referred to as GBE, or ginkgo biloba extract. Most standardized products contain 22 to 27 percent ginkgo flavone glycosides (or flavonoids) and 5 to 7 percent terpene lactones. Standardized GBE is also available in liquid form, with 9.6 milligrams flavone glycosides and 2.4 milligrams terpene lactones per dose.

Each type of commercial preparation has its advantages and disadvantages. The following summary can help you understand the uses of various forms of ginkgo.

TEAS OR INFUSIONS

Teas are probably the oldest form of medicinal herb preparation and are the traditional way to use ginkgo over a period of months. A tea is more formally known as an infusion; to prepare an infusion, the herb is steeped in hot water. A decoction is like an infusion, only it is prepared using boiling water.

Infusions and decoctions tend to work quickly in the body. The hot or boiling water extracts the most important active ingredients in ginkgo, making them easier for the body to absorb. The Chinese have used ginkgo tea for centuries in the treatment of asthma and bronchitis.

Unfortunately, ginkgo tea can have a bit-

TEA TIME

To prepare gingko tea, put 1 ounce dried leaves into 2 cups water. Simmer over low heat for five minutes. Let it cool, then strain and drink ¼ cup warm twice a day.

---

ter, slightly sour, astringent flavor, which many people find unpleasant. You might be able to overcome some of these unpleasant flavors by adding lemon, honey or sugar as well as aromatic herbs (such as chamomile or peppermint) to the tea.

TINCTURES AND LIQUID EXTRACTS

There are two main types of extracts or tinctures—alcohol-based and glycerin-based products. Of the two, the vast majority of ginkgo products sold are alcohol extracts. (Most glycerin extracts are given to children and to people who should avoid ethyl alcohol.)

To use a liquid extract, put forty drops in a little warm water or juice and drink morning, midday, and evening, as needed.

To prepare your own tincture or alcohol extract, crush up the dried ginkgo leaves to form four to eight ounces of coarse powder. Place the powder in a Mason jar and cover it with sixteen ounces of 80-proof vodka or with ¾ cup of Everclear and 1 ¼ cups of water. Mark the jar with the date, then tuck it away in a cool, dark place. Don't forget about it; you'll need to shake it well every day. After two weeks, strain the mixture or pour it through a coffee filter to remove the sediment. Store the finished extract in amber bottles away from heat and sunlight. Date the bottle; the extract should be good for up to three years.

POWDERS, CAPSULES, AND TABLETS

Many people find it easier to use ginkgo after the leaves have been ground into a powder. Powdered ginkgo is sold as capsules, tablets, or a loose powder (which can be formed into capsules).

Powdered ginkgo can be concentrated and standardized. A typical dose of standardized powdered ginkgo extract is one 40-milligram tablet three times daily. Look for a product standardized to 24 percent ginko flavoglycosides and 6 percent terpene lactones, the ratios used in most scientific studies.

GROW YOUR OWN GINKGO

The ginkgo tree is a beautiful addition to any landscaping plan—and the wedge- or

BEYOND THE LEAVES

Most modern herbalists use only ginkgo leaves in their preparations, but the ancient Chinese used the nuts (also called the fruit) and the seeds as well. After they have been cooked, they are said to taste like giant pine nuts.

The nuts, which look like plums and mature in late fall, contain terpenes that irritate the skin and cause painful digestive spasms if eaten. The Chinese boil the nuts to remove the terpenes, then add them to soups and stews. As a general rule, it is best to avoid contact with ginkgo nuts since about one out of three people develop a severe rash after handling the plant.

fan-shape leaves can be used as medicine throughout the year. Ginkgo trees lose their leaves each fall; these leaves can be harvested and used to make herbal preparations.

The ginkgo tree is grown across most of the United States; it does well as far north as eastern Massachusetts and central Michigan. It grows in many cities, where it has earned a reputation as a beautiful and hearty tree, because it can withstand attacks from insects, fungi, pollution, and other destructive forces.

Ginkgo trees come in male and female forms; the males produce slender, stalked flowers known as catkins, while the females form the fruits. When used as ornamental trees, many people prefer males, since the fruit of the female tree can cause skin irritation and it smells like rancid butter. (The fruit or nut of the female tree contains an irritating chemical similar to that found in poison ivy and poison oak.)

To grow a ginkgo tree from seeds, place the seeds in moist sand inside a plastic bag for several months and store in the refrigerator. In the spring, take them out and plant them in a good potting mixture. Be sure the soil contains plenty of nitrogen to optimize growth.

Ginkgo trees grow very slowly for the first twenty years or so, reaching a height of about twenty to thirty feet. As the tree comes of age, its limbs become heavier, fuller, and they spread out. They can reach a height of eighty to one hundred feet and a width of twenty feet, but this type of growth can take hundreds of years. Very old trees can have trunks as much as eight feet in diameter. Ginkgo trees can live for more than 1,000 years, providing centuries of beauty and healing benefits.

The trees fan-shaped leaves, which have many parallel veins, reach two or three inches across; they are not like the leaves of any other flowering trees. The leaves resemble the leaves of the maidenhair fern, which is one of the reasons the plant is called the maidenhair tree.

There are four main types of ginkgo trees:

- *Fastigiata:* A tree with a columnar form that has almost erect branches

- *Macrophylla laciniata*: A tree with larger leaves than *Ginkgo fastigiata*

- *Pendula:* A tree with drooping or weeping branches

- *Variegata:* A tree with variegated leaves of pale-yellow streaks through green.

All of the trees appear to share similar medicinal effects; select a type that you find most aesthetically pleasing.

The best time to harvest the ginkgo leaves is in the late summer (late August or September), just before they begin to change color and turn golden yellow. The flavonoids, ginkgolides, bilobalides, and other active ingredients reach their peak at this time.

After picking the leaves, allow them to dry in the shade by placing them on a screen so that they can have good air circulation from the top and bottom. Ideally, they should dry in two or three days without becoming overheated or being exposed to direct sun. The leaves are sufficiently dry if they snap when bent. Store the dried leaves

A ONE-BRANCHED FAMILY TREE

Ginkgo biloba is the sole representative of the genus Ginkgo, in the family Ginkgoaceae, order Ginkgoales, class Gymnospermae. It is more closely related to pines and other cone-producing trees (conifers) than it is to so-called angiosperm trees, such as maples and oaks.

in a paper bag inside a plastic bag kept in a cool, dark place. The dried leaves can be used to prepare teas or infusions (see page 155) or tinctures (see page 156).

CHAPTER 9

Designing Your Ginkgo Program

By now you know that ginkgo biloba can strengthen your circulatory system, enhance brain function, reverse impotence, improve vision and hearing, and help to treat other health problems as well. You know that ginkgo has been used safely for thousands of years as a natural remedy and that it is free of many of the unwanted side effects associated with traditional pharmaceutical drugs.

Even if you are intrigued by the possibilities of using ginkgo to help manage your particular health problems, you may still hesitate to try the herb because you are not sure how to use it safely and effectively. This chapter will help you design a ginkgo treatment program to meet your individual needs.

While ginkgo has an impressive record in both safety and efficacy, it should be used only with the approval of your doctor or health care provider. According to one recent survey, three out of four people who took herbal supplements said that they did not tell their doctor about the herbs; this is an unwise and potentially unsafe practice. Your doctor needs to be aware of all medications and supplements you are taking, even if you believe that they are safe.

Self-treatment with ginkgo (or any other herb, for that matter) is not recommended for serious brain, heart, or circulatory problems. If you experience impotence, changes in vision, or hearing loss, check with your doctor before using ginkgo to reverse the symptoms. These problems can be symptoms of a more serious systemic health problem. In all cases, let your doctor know that you are interested in using ginkgo as part of your treatment plan.

Sometimes you may need to educate your physician about the use of ginkgo and other herbal treatments. If your doctor objects to the use of herbs as part of your overall approach to health, ask whether this is an uninformed decision or one based on scientific research. In other words, find out if there is a specific and justified reason for you to avoid taking ginkgo, or whether your doctor is simply ignorant of the many benefits associated with using the herb.

IS GINKGO RIGHT FOR YOU?

Ginkgo biloba extract is considered nontoxic when used internally; it is virtually free of all unwanted side effects. According to research, it can be used safely with other supplements without interaction and has no reported toxicity. In fact, in more than forty-four research trials involving 9,772 study participants, no serious problems were reported, even among people who took as much as 600 milligrams ginkgo per dose. Of the people in the studies, fewer than 1 percent in this sample had mild stomach upset or occasional headaches. No one reported any drug interactions, although many of the people in the study were using other drugs or herbs as well. In another 1988 study, only 33 of 8,505 patients taking ginkgo biloba reported mild unwanted side effects, typically gastrointestinal upset.

NOTE: While ginkgo may not cause unwanted side effects, it can thin the blood, so it is not recommended for people with clotting disorders or for those taking aspirin or other blood-thinning drugs, such as warfarin (Coumadin and Parwarfin), streptokinase (Streptase), and urokinase (Abbokinase), among others. If you take vitamin E or garlic, both natural supplements known to inhibit platelet stickiness, discuss the use of ginkgo with your doctor, who may want to perform a clotting test to monitor your clotting time.

The pulp of the fruit of the ginkgo tree can produce severe contact dermatitis and other allergic skin reactions in many people. This is of no relevance to you if you plan to use commercially prepared ginkgo products. However, if you have a ginkgo tree in your yard or if you encounter one in a public area, avoid skin contact with the fleshy part of the fruit.

MAKING GINKGO WORK FOR YOU

If you would like to use ginkgo to support your circulatory system and improve your overall health, you must learn how to use the herb safely and effectively. The following questions will guide you through many of the common decisions you must make as you customize your ginkgo program.

How much ginkgo should I take?

The standard dose of ginkgo biloba extract tablets used in most clinical studies is 40 milligrams standardized extract three times per day (120 milligrams a day) over a period of at least eight weeks. In some studies, people have taken twice that amount— 80 milligrams three times a day or 240 milligrams a day—with success.

Most preparations are taken three times a day, but some products are designed to be used only twice daily. Follow the package directions on the product you are using. Because ginkgo is an exceptionally safe herb, using it in higher amounts should not cause any adverse health effects, although it can be a waste of money if you take more herb that your body needs.

How long until I see results?

Most people see improvement in their health after using ginkgo for eight to twelve weeks; however, in some cases it may take up to twenty-four weeks (six months). Researchers theorize that a slow response may indicate that certain areas of the brain have long been deprived of oxygen and nutrients, so they respond to treatment and revitalize more slowly. For example, a twelve-week French study of people with vertigo found noticeable improvement in balance after thirty days and significant improvement after sixty days, with still more impressive results after ninety days.

Do I need to take ginkgo on an ongoing basis?

Research indicates that ginkgo can be effective, even when taken periodically.

For example, a study done on the workers who cleaned up the Chernobyl nuclear plant found that the beneficial effects of ginkgo use lasted for seven months, even when people stopped using ginkgo after the twelve-week study period. This study indicates that you may be able to enjoy the health benefits of ginkgo without the expense of taking the herb on an ongoing basis. One approach would be to use it daily for two to three months, discontinue use for one or two months, then repeat the cycle. Again, taking the herb on a continual basis would have no known adverse health consequences, although it could be an unnecessary expense if the additional herb is not providing any meaningful health benefits.

When should I start taking ginkgo?

Do not wait until you experience the ravages of growing older to begin using the herb. According to ancient Chinese practice and many modern herbalists, people should start taking ginkgo in their late teens or twenties to prevent circulatory problems and other conditions associated with aging. Assuming there are no health reasons to prevent you from taking the herb, the only disincentive involves the cost of using ginkgo; this is a trade-off that must be considered by the individual. You might try taking 120 milligrams ginkgo daily for three months, then assess how you feel.

Should I take ginkgo any particular time of day?

Ginkgo is most effective when it is taken in regular doses and, if possible, at the same times every day. Studies have found that the levels of ginkgo in the body peak about one hour after taking the herb. To maintain a more consistent level of herb in your system, take the ginkgo in divided doses throughout the day.

Can ginkgo help prevent damage caused by radiation exposure?

Yes. If you have been exposed to excessive ultraviolet radiation from the sun—whether you have a sunburn or not—it is prudent to take ginkgo to help the body manage the stress caused by the exposure. For the same reason, it can be helpful to take ginkgo after exposure to X rays.

Should I look for a standardized ginkgo product?

Most commercial ginkgo products are standardized extracts. Many of the best-selling commercial products are standardized to a 24 percent content of flavone glycosides; in other words, the products are processed so that they contain a specific, fixed amount of active ingredients to maximize the medicinal effect of the herb. Most of the clinical trials have used these standardized extracts.

Without standardization, the active ingredients in ginkgo can vary by as much as 200 percent, depending on the growing conditions, the location, the time of year the leaves were harvested, and how they were handled during the production process. Despite the variation in intensity, some herbalists favor the use of unstandardized products because they do not interfere with the natural balance of the herb. With unstandardized products, the ingredients occur in the extract just as they do in the whole plant. Some herbalists also object to the use of ginkgo extracts as a medicine used to treat symptoms of disease rather than as a tonic used to strengthen the body as a whole.

As a general rule, you might want to use standardized ginkgo products when taking the herb to address specific health problems, such as a circulatory problem or hearing impairment. If, however, you plan to use ginkgo as a preventive measure, you may want to opt for a whole-plant, unstandardized extract.

Which form of ginkgo is best?

Most herbalists recommend the use of liquid extracts over powdered capsules or tablets because they tend to be more potent. Concentrated powdered extracts can also be effective, and they are quite popular in Europe and Japan.

Can ginkgo be combined with other herbs?

Yes, ginkgo often is combined with many other herbs, depending on the condition being treated. The herbs that share the healing properties of ginkgo are listed in the previous chapters; for example, other herbs helpful in enhancing memory and brain function are discussed in Chapter 3.

In traditional Chinese medicine, ginkgo is used with as many as ten or twelve different herbs to create a blended formula customized to an individual's particular needs. Common herbs used in combination with ginkgo include: astragalus (*Astragalus membranaceus*), Butcher's broom (*Ruscus aculeatus*), cayenne (*Capsicum frutescens*), dandelion (*Taraxacum officinale*), echinacea (*Echinacea angustifolia*), garlic (*Allium sativum*), ginseng (*Panax ginseng, P.*

quinquefolius, or *P. sentocosus*),
goldenseal (*Hydrastis canadensis*), gotu
kola (*Centella asiatica*), and rosemary
(*Rosmarinus officinalis*).

Many so-called brain enhancing
herbal formulas combine some or all of
these ingredients, as well as additional
vitamins, minerals, and amino acids. As
a general rule, avoid these products
unless you know the product's exact
ingredients so that you can be assured of
its contents and efficacy.

Organizations of Interest

**American Association of Naturopathic
Physicians**
601 Valley Street
Suite 105
Seattle, WA 98109
(206) 298-0125
www.naturopathic.org

This association can provide referrals to naturopathic physicians who are members. In addition, the group offers brochures and background information on naturopathic medicine.

American Botanical Council
P.O. Box 144345
Austin, TX 78714-4345
(512) 331-8868

(800) 373-7105

www.herbalgram.org

This nonprofit educational organization is dedicated to providing information on herbs to practitioners of herbal medicine and the public. It also publishes the quarterly journal, *HerbalGram*, which is readable but with a strongly scientific focus. Cost: $25 per year.

American Herb Association

P.O. Box 1673

Nevada City, CA 95959

(530) 265-9552

The association provides its members with a quarterly newsletter that includes updates on current studies, reviews of books and videos, and legal news and controversies regarding herbs. It also offers directories of mail-order herb products.

Herb Research Foundation
1007 Pearl Street
Suite 200
Boulder, CO 80302
(303) 449-2265
www.herbs.org

The foundation is a medicinal library that provides packets of information about individual herbs, including ginkgo. Standard information packets cost $7 for nonmembers or $5 for members. The foundation does not sell herbs.

Institute for Traditional Medicine
2017 Southeast Hawthorne
Portland, OR 97214
(503) 233-4907
www.europa.com/~itm

The nonprofit institute provides educational materials and conducts research on natural healing for health professionals and interested consumers.

Qi-Gong Institute/East-West Academy of Healing Arts
450 Sutter Street
San Francisco, CA 94108
(415) 788-2227

The academy is a nonprofit corporation founded in 1973. It is dedicated to educating, training, and healing people using the 5,000-year-old traditional form of Chinese energy medicine known as Qigong. The academy holds classes and seminars and publishes material on Qigong and complementary alternative medicine.

Mail-Order Sources of Herbs

Blessed Herbs
109 Barrie Plains Road
Oakham, MA 01068
(800) 489-4372

Dabney Herbs
P.O. Box 22061
Lewisville, KY 40252
(502) 893-5198
www.dabneyherbs.com

Earth's Harvest
14385 S.E. Lusted Road
Sandy, OR 97055
(800) 428-3308

East Earth Trade Winds
P.O. Box 493151
Redding, CA 96049-3151

(800) 258-6878
(916) 241-6878 in California
(800) 258-1384
www.snowcrest.net/eetw/

Eclectic Institute
14385 Lusted Road
Sandy, OR 97055
(800) 332-HERB
www.eclecticherb.com

Gardens of the Blue Ridge
P.O. Box 10
Pineola, NC 28662
(704) 733-2417

Great China Herb Company
857 Washington Street
San Francisco, CA 94108
(415) 982-2195

Herb-Pharm
P.O. Box 116
William, OR 97544
(503) 846-6262

Herbs Etc.
1345 Cerrillos Road
Santa Fe, NM 87505
(800) 634-3727

Herbs of Grace
Division of School of Natural Medicine
P.O. Box 7369
Boulder, CO 80306-7369
(303) 455-8048
www.purehealth.com

Institute for Traditional Medicine
2017 S.E. Hawthorne
Portland, OR 97214
(800) 544-7504
www.europa.com/~itm

Mayway U.S.A.
1338 Mandela Parkway
Oakland, CA 94607
(510) 208-3113
www.mayway.com

McZand Herbal Inc.
P.O. Box 5312
Santa Monica, CA 90409
(310) 822-0500
(800) 800-0405
www.zand.com

Meridian Traditional Herbal Products
44 Linden Street
Brookline, MA 02146
(800) 356-6003
(617) 739-2636 in Massachusetts

Nature's Way Products, Inc.
10 Mountain Springs Parkway
Springville, UT 84663
(801) 489-1520
www.naturesway.com

Rainbow Light
207 McPherson Street
Santa Cruz, CA 95060
(800) 635-1233
(800) 227-0555

Turtle Island Herbs
1705 14th Street, No. 172
Boulder, CO 80302
(303) 442-2215

White Crane
426 First Street
Jersey City, NJ 07302
(800) 994-3721

Windriver Herbs
P.O. Box 3876
Jackson, WY 83001
(800) 903-HERB

Wise Woman Herbals
P.O. Box 279
Creswell, OR 97426
(800) 532-5219

Web Sites of Interest

Other Web sites of interest are included in the list of organizations of interest on page 179.

Algy's Herb Page:
www.algy.com/herb/index.html

The Alternative Medicine Homepage:
www.pitt.edu/~cbw/altm.html

HealthGate:
www.healthgate.com

Institute for Traditional Medicine:
www.europa.com/~itm

MedWeb:
www.medweb.emory.edu

Yahoo!'s Alternative Medicine Page:
www.yahoo.com/health/
alternative__medicine

Yahoo! Health: Women's Health:
**www.yahoo.com/health/women_s_
health**

Bibliography

BOOKS

Halpern, Georges. *Ginkgo: A Practical Guide.* Garden City, NY: Avery Publishing Group, 1998.

Hobbs, Christopher. *Ginkgo: Elixir of Youth.* Loveland, CO: Botanica Press, 1991.

McClain, Gary. *The Natural Way of Healing Asthma and Allergies.* New York: Dell, 1995.

Murray, Frank. *Ginkgo Biloba.* New Canaan, CT: Keats Publishing, 1996.

———. *Ginkgo Biloba: The Amazing 200 million-year-old healer.* New Canaan, CT.: Keats Publishing, 1993.

Murray, Michael T. *Male Sexual Vitality.* Rocklin, CA: Prima Publishing, 1994.

Murray, Michael T., and Pizzorno, J. *Encyclopedia of Natural Medicine*. Rocklin, CA: Prima Publishing, 1991.

Peterson, Nicola. *Ginkgo & Garlic: Natural Remedies for Respiratory and Circulatory Problems*. London: Souvenir Press, 1998.

Pizzorno, J., and Murray, M., eds. *A Textbook of Natural Medicine*. Seattle, WA: Bastyr College Publications, 1991.

Rothfeld, Glenn S., and LeVert, Suzanne. *Ginkgo Biloba*. New York: Dell, 1998.

Tenney, Louise. *Ginkgo*. Pleasant Grove, UT: Woodland Publishing, 1996.

ARTICLES

Attella, M. J., et al. "Ginkgo Biloba Extract Facilitates Recovery from Penetrating Brain Injury in Adult Male Rats." *Exp. Neurol* 105 (1989): 62–71.

Bauer, U. "6-Month Double-Blind Randomized Clinical Trial of Ginkgo Biloba Extract Versus

Placebo in Two Parallel Groups in Patients Suffering from Peripheral Arterial Insufficiency." *Arzneim. Forsch* 34 (1984): 716.

Becker, L. E., and Skipworth, G. B. "Ginkgo-tree dermatitis, Stomatitis, and Procitis." *Journal of the American Medical Association* 231 (1975): 1162.

Brown, Donald J. "Ginkgo Biloba—Old and New: Part II." *Let's Live* 5 (May 1992): 62–64.

Chesseboeuf, L., et al. "Comparative Study of Two Vasoregulators in Syndromes of Deafness and Vertigo." *Medicine du Nord et de l'Est*, 5 (1979): 534.

Courbier R., et al. "Double-Blind, Cross-Over Study of Tanakan in Arterial Diseases of the Legs." *Mediterranee Medicale* 126 (1977): 61–64.

Duke, M. V., and Salni, M. L. "Purification and Characterization of an Iron-Containing Superoxide Dismutase from a Eukaryote, Ginkgo Biloba." *Archives of Biochem. Biophys* 243 (1985): 305–314.

Evans, D. A., et al. "Clinically-Diagnosed Alzheimer's Disease: An Epidemiological Study in a Community Population of Older Persons." *Journal of the American Medical Association*, November 10, 1989.

Foster, Steven. "Ginkgo Biloba: A Living Fossil for Today's Health Needs." *Better Nutrition* 4 (April 1996): 59.

Gaby, Alan R., and Wright, Jonathan V. "Nutritional Factors in Degenerative Eye Disorders: Cataract and Macular Degeneration." *Journal of the Advancement of Medicine* 6 (Spring 1993): 27–40.

Gebner, B., and Klasser, M. "Study of the Long-Term Action of Ginkgo Biloba Extract on Vigilance and Mental Performance as Determined by Means of Quantitative Pharmaco-EEG and Psychometric Measurements." *Arzneim-Forsch*. 35 (1985): 1459–1465.

Goldberg, Jack, et al. "Factors Associated With Age-Related Macular Degeneration." *Ameri-*

can Journal of Epidemiology 128 (1988): 700–710.

Guinot, P., et al. "Effect of BN 52063, a Specific PAF-Acether Antagonist, on Bronchial Provocation Test to Allergen in Asthmatic Patients. A Preliminary Study." *Prostaglandins* 34 (1987): 723–731.

Guinot, P., et al. "Treatment of Adult Systemic Mastocytosis with a PAF-Acether Antagonist BN52063." *Lancet* 11 (1988): 114.

Hindmarch, I., and Subhan, Z. "The Psychopharmacological Effects of Ginkgo Biloba Extract in Normal Healthy Volunteers." *Int. J. Clin. Pharmacol. Res.* 35 (1984): 89–93.

Holger, K. M., Axelsson, A., and Pringle, I. "Ginkgo Biloba Extract for the Treatment of Tinnitus." *Audiology* 33 (1994): 85–92.

Kleijnen, J., and Knipschild, P. "Ginkgo Biloba for Cerebral Insufficiency." *British Journal of Clinical Pharmacology* 34 (1992): 352–358.

Koltringer, P., et al. "Ginkgo Biloba Extract and Folic Acid in the Treatment of Autonomic Neuropathies." *Acta Medica Austriaca* 16 (1989): 35–37.

Koltringer, P., et al. "Ginkgo Biloba Special Extract EGb 761 and Folic Acid in Diabetic Neuropathia, a Randomized, Placebo-Controlled, Double-Blind Study." *Z. Allg. Med* 68 (1992): 69–102.

Kurosawa, M., et al. "Increased Levels of Blood Platelet-Activating Factor in Bronchial Asthmatic Patients with Active Symptoms." *Allergy* 49 (1994): 60–63.

Lebuisson, D. A., et al. "Treatment of Senile Macular Degeneration with Ginkgo Biloba Extract: A Preliminary Double-Blind Study Versus Placebo." *Presse Med* 15 (1986): 1556–1558.

Meyer, B. "A Multicenter Randomized Double-Blind Study of Ginkgo Biloba Extract Versus Placebo in the Treatment of Tinnitus." *Presse Med* 15 (1986): 1562–1564.

Rai, G. S., Shovlin, C., and Wesnes, K. A. "A Double-Blind, Placebo-Controlled Study of Ginkgo Biloba Extract ("Tanakan") in Elderly Outpatients with Mild to Moderate Memory Impairment." *Current Medical Research and Opinion* 12 (1991): 350–354.

Root, Elizabeth J., and Longenecker, John B. "Nutrition, the Brain and Alzheimer's Disease." *Nutrition Today* (July–August 1988): 11–18.

Schilcher, H. "Ginkgo Biloba: Investigation on the Quality, Activity, Effectiveness, and Safety." *Zeit. F. Phytother* 9 (1988): 119–127.

Sikora, R., et al. "Ginkgo Biloba Extract in the Treatment of Erectile Dysfunction." *Journal of Urology* 141 (1989): 188A.

Smith, P. F., Maclennan K., and Darlington, C. L. "The Neuroprotective Properties of the Ginkgo Biloba Leaf: A Review of the Possible Relationship to Platelet-Activating Factor (PAF)." *Journal of Ethnopharmacology* 50 (1996): 131–139.

Sprenger, F. H. "Inner Ear Hearing Loss—Good Results with Ginkgo Biloba." *Ztl. Praxis* 38 (1986): 938–940.

Taillandier, J., et al. "Treatment of Cerebral Disorders Due to Aging with Ginkgo Biloba Extract. Longitudinal, Multicentre, Double-Blind Study Versus Placebo." *Presse Med* 15 (1986): 1583–1587.

Tamborini, A., and Taurelle, R. "Value of Standardized Ginkgo Biloba Extract (EGb 761) in the Management of Congestive Symptoms of Premenstrual Syndrome." *Review Gynecol. Obstet* 88 (July–September 1993): 447–457.

Vorberg, G. "Ginkgo Biloba Extract (GBE): A Long-Term Study of Chronic Cerebral Insufficiency in Geriatric Patients." *Clinical Trials Journal* 22 (1985): 149–157.

Wesnes, K., et al. "A Double-Blind Placebo-Based Trial of Tanakan in the Treatment of Idiopathic Cognitive Impairment in the Elderly." *Human Psychopharmacology* 2 (1987): 159–169.

About the Author

Winifred Conkling is a freelance writer specializing in health and consumer topics. She is the author of more than fifteen books on natural medicine and health, including *Secrets of Ginseng, Secrets of Enchinacea, Secrets of 5-HTP, Natural Healing for Children*, and *Natural Remedies for Arthritis*. Her work has been published in a number of national magazines, including *American Health, Consumer Reports, McCall's*, and *Reader's Digest*. She lives in northern Virginia with her husband and two children.